# Dancing for Health

# Dancing for Health

## Conquering and Preventing Stress

Judith Lynne Hanna

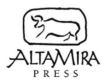

**ALTAMIRA**
PRESS

A Division of
ROWMAN & LITTLEFIELD PUBLISHERS, INC.
*Lanham • New York • Toronto • Oxford*

ALTAMIRA PRESS
A division of Rowman & Littlefield Publishers, Inc.
A wholly owned subsidary of The Rowman & Littlefield Publishing Group, Inc.
4501 Forbes Boulevard, Suite 200
Lanham, MD 20706
www.altamirapress.com

PO Box 317, Oxford OX2 9RU, UK

British Library Cataloguing in Publication Information Available

**Library of Congress Cataloging-in-Publication Data**

Hanna, Judith Lynne.
    Dancing for health : conquering and preventing stress / Judith Lynne Hanna.
        p.   cm.
    Rev. ed. of: Dance and stress. New York : AMS Press, c1988.
    Includes bibliographical references and index.
    ISBN-13: 978-0-7591-0859-2 (pbk. : alk. paper)
    ISBN-10: 0-7591-0859-5 (pbk. : alk. paper)
        1. Dance—Psychological aspects.   2. Stress (Psychology)   3. Dance therapy.
    I. Hanna, Judith Lynne. Dance and stress.   II. Title.

    GV1588.5.H36 2006
    793.301′9—dc22
                                                                        2006002758

Printed in the United States of America

∞™ The paper used in this publication meets the minimum requirements of American National Standard for Information Sciences—Permanence of Paper for Printed Library Materials, ANSI/NISO Z39.48-1992.

~

# Contents

~

# Acknowledgments

A book is the result of an author's exchanges with other people. Among these whom I wish to thank for their help with this book and for generously sharing resources and observations are Ruth and John Solomon, Don L. F. Nilsen, Robyn Cruz, and Gillian Ice. The University of Maryland libraries have continually offered multiple services. William John Hanna, my always-helpful colleague, assisted with computer production of the text and images. I thank Chris Dame for graciously allowing me to include many of his fine photographs. I appreciate Anya Peterson Royce introducing me to Mitch Allen, former AltaMira publisher and editor. I owe a special debt to Allen, who not only supported this publication but shared with me some of his experiences as a dancer with ethnic dance companies (Aman and others) for a couple of decades.

# PART I

# SETTING THE STAGE

Life is stressful. We face unending horrific man-made and natural disasters as well as lesser provocations. Three out of four Americans complain of chronic stress. People call out for healing. Like a diamond with radiant facets, dance attracts our attention, feels good to do, and has the potential to meet our needs for stress relief and good health. Dance is a means to resist, reduce, and escape stress. How do we know? Through time and across space, humans have turned to dance for self-protection. Current health research is telling. Yet dance can also induce stress.

What's in your head? What's in your body? What role does culture play? The concepts of stress, dance, and their connections lay the groundwork for our itinerary.

# Prelude

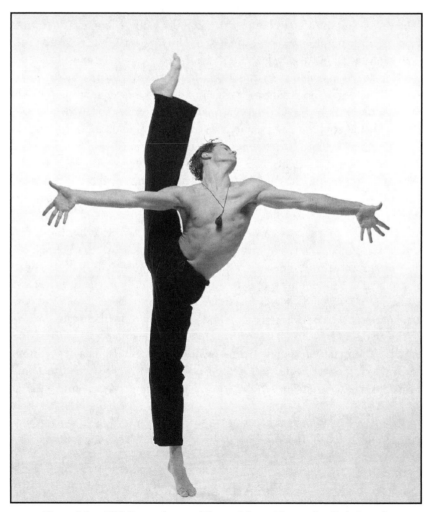

**Figure P.1.   9/11 Remembrance (Photo of Rasta Thomas by Chris Dame)**

## 9/11

September 11, 2001. Horrific unprecedented terrorism on United States soil. Nearly three thousand people gruesomely killed at the World Trade Center in New York City as two hijacked American planes crashed into the majestic Twin Towers. People from eighty countries lost their lives. Terrorists also flew an American plane to Pennsylvania, where passengers forced the plane to crash into a field to avoid hitting an unknown target. All aboard died. Terrorists crashed a fourth plane into the Pentagon in Washington, D.C., reducing one of its walls to a pile of rubbish. Yet more deaths. A militant Muslim sect, seeking to impose its worldview all over the planet and ensure political control, targeted symbols of American power, modernity, and the global economy. Westerners have been demonized and said to be deserving of death. Electrified by bold air assaults and long inspired by Bin Laden's rhetoric, money, and example, al Qaeda now counts among its members Islamic radicals worldwide for whom sympathy is felt among millions of Muslims. And then the mysterious deadly anthrax mailings in the United States killed five innocents, made eighteen others ill, and contaminated numerous government buildings, disrupting the U.S. Congress. Culprit of the bioterrorist attack unidentified and still at large. A passenger aboard another U.S. airplane was discovered with a bomb in his shoe. The war in Iraq, hostage taking, beheading, and destruction continue.

Although many potential threats worldwide have been thwarted, terrorism occurs and threats persist. For the first time in its history, the United States faces a different kind of enemy embedded in webs and networks of terrorism spread across about sixty nations. From a comfortable existence before 9/11, Americans were thrust into a new and unfamiliar world. Living with low-level unpredictable vulnerability, they have become exiles from the secure past of endless prosperity and safety from foreign attack. As citizens of the most powerful nation in the world, Americans find it hard to fathom their vulnerability.

Survivors and the rest of the nation cried out for healing. The sheer scale of 9/11 has dwarfed professional mental health resources.[1] Trauma experts were in demand. Mental health practitioners continued to be needed in family assistance centers, offices, schools, stadia having memorial events, medical and psychiatric hospitals, clinics, and communities. The emotional force was so strong that even people accustomed to coping on their own sought help, and people may not come forward to work through the trauma for years.

## The Arts and Healing

Following 9/11, the Arts Partnership (U.S. Department of Education, National Endowment for the Arts, state arts alliances, and other arts organizations nationwide) and Americans for the Arts called attention to the role of the arts in healing, recovery, and rebuilding both self and community. The experience of distress cries out for a means to manage it, to resist, reduce, or escape. Emotional wrenching requires healing. Psyches need rebuilding. Communities seek renewal. And people seek comfort in the arts and their restorative powers. After the first stunned reaction to the tragedy of 9/11, theater historian Marvin Carlson reports, the theater community "rallied, and in reaction to the strategies of the administration's 'war on terror,' began to produce the most concentrated and dedicated political theater to appear in America since the 1960s . . . most concentrated in the Off- and Off-Off Broadway theaters of New York."[2]

In the Judeo-Christian tradition, the arts are deemed relevant to the process of healing. Beginning in the 1970s, Charles Leslie, pioneer in medical anthropology, recognized the power of the aesthetic, symbolic, and performative dimensions of healing.[3] In the increasingly multicultural United States, people from all continents bring with them their spiritual beliefs and traditional practices in the arts of healing. Some transformation often occurs, but so do retentions. Traditional nonindustrial societies have often collectivized the response to stress with healing rituals and religious ceremonies that include dance.

Responding to 9/11, the Los Angeles public forum on Arts and Health at the City of Hope National Medical Center invited me, in my capacity as an anthropologist and dance educator, to discuss how dance can help individuals manage stress. Since dance, a language-like form of human culture, has psychobiological dynamics, I have over the years engaged the relevant fields of cultural, linguistic, physical, psychological, applied, and medical anthropology.[4] The Postgraduate Center for Mental Health; Johns Hopkins University Public Health Program; Uniformed Services University of Health Sciences, School of Medicine; and the National Symposium on Pain are among the institutions in the United States and abroad that have invited me to speak and exchange ideas on dance and health.

So 9/11 was the catalyst to rewrite my book *Dance and Stress: Resistance, Reduction and Euphoria*, published in 1988 in a series called Stress in Modern Society and apparently the first work to explore broadly the dance-stress connection. Since early history, humans have danced to cope with stress. Dance is one of several approaches that contribute to healing, although the pursuit of a dance career has stressor elements, for example, competition, stage fright, physical injury, racism, economic difficulties, and career transition. Dance is like a diamond with radiant facets. It is fascinating to look at, and it is highly valued for its instrumental hardness. In this book, I draw upon knowledge about dance, stress, and the connections between the two that have come to the fore over the past two decades.

## Anxious Times

Anxious times cause stress, a response to adversities or challenges in a person's life. However, your own psychology, interpersonal support, constraints, opportunities, and culture mediate stress. Meanings and values, at the center of human life, represent the essence of stress, emotion, and adaptation. Cultural sensibility can distinguish what a group perceives as normal developments from the problematic.

Emotional distress is a normal response to horrific events. We feel ripples of tragedy and uncertainty, shock and sadness, fear and helplessness, and it is possible for these events to result in stress disorder, a pathological response called post-traumatic stress syndrome that interferes with functioning. Pathology lies not in the symptoms—a normal reaction to stress—but in the persistence of the symptoms and the amount of distress they cause. A victim can be overwhelmed by multiple problems arising from a single event. Symptoms of post-traumatic stress disorder include reliving the trauma; mental flashbacks; sleepless nights; nightmares; irritability; overindulgence in work, drugs, or food; dissociation and distancing from intimates; nonspecific ailments;

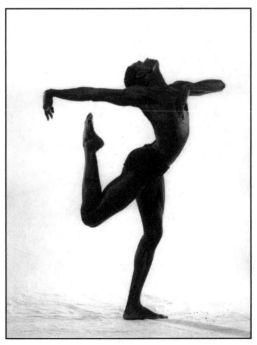

**Figure P.2.  Stressed (Photo of Oscar Hawkins by Chris Dame)**

depression; acting out; startle responses; withdrawal; fearfulness; anxiety; out-breaks of rage; trembling; ticks; aversion to body parts or bodily functions; high levels of forgetfulness; altering identity; and repetitive behavior.

Based on an army survey of about six thousand American soldiers and marines engaged in ground combat operations in Iraq in 2003, researchers found that these troops developed more mental health problems (16 percent) than those soldiers on the ground in Afghanistan in 2002 (11 percent). Af-ter duty, major depression and anxiety disorder stemmed from being shot at; handling dead bodies; knowing someone who was injured or killed, killing an enemy combatant; close calls, such as having been saved from being wounded by wearing body armor; sights of death and destruction; smells of burned flesh; and sounds of wailing mothers searching for their miss-ing children among debris. The army researchers are taking a proactive approach to identifying mental health problems in returning soldiers from Iraq in particular. Psychiatrists learned only years after soldiers returned from Vietnam that many of them had post-traumatic stress disorder, which delayed treatment.[5] The psychological strain of war elicits stressful moral questions: Could the loss of friends and the unintentional killing of civilians have been avoided?

Of course, there have been and will continue to be other kinds of trauma worldwide in which the past cohabits with the present: political persecution, torture, imprisonment, organized violence including mass and public raping at the hands of both government and opposition forces (psychologically dev-astating to a parent as protector and to the value of virginity and the sign of a woman's fidelity), counterinsurgency campaigns, ethnic cleansing, com-bustible disagreements over means of conflict resolution, involuntary migra-tion, abusive parents and sexual partners, gang clashes, organized crime, police brutality, serial killers, sexual assault, and race and gender discrimination. The twentieth century brought some of the most barbaric episodes of efficiently organized large-scale violence and trauma: the Holocaust, Cambodian killing fields, Stalin's slaughter, ethnic cleansing in the former Yugoslavia, and blood-baths in Rwanda, Burundi, and Sudan. Such traumas often lead to refugee and runaway situations or other kinds of homelessness.

The impact of stress may be indelible. As a volunteer for the Victim As-sistance Sexual Assault Program of Montgomery County, Maryland, I met a distraught mother whose teenage daughter had been raped. She told me that she herself had been kidnapped at ten years of age, along with her three-year-old brother, while her family was in Vietnam. The Vietnamese put her in a hole and periodically raped her until she was rescued; she now avoids all Asians: "I see their slit eyes and panic."

An unending list of stressors appears in the news. When one confronts change, such as residential relocation, it is often difficult to avoid stress. Social and cultural stressors include poverty, anarchy, U.S. government credibility and deadlock, partisan disorder, an economy hemorrhaging jobs and business failure, erosion of civil liberties and social supports developed in the aftermath of the 1929 Depression, disjunction between aspirations and ability or opportunity, pollution of air and water, unsafe drugs on the market, gentrification and destruction of all or part of your emotional ecosystem, and valorization of deviance. Identity of race, ethnicity, sexual orientation, religion, politics, gender, age—and identity theft—can be stressors. Corporate world scandals at WorldCom, Enron, and other businesses; pedophilia in the Catholic church; parental expectations;[6] teen suicide; last-minute preparation for holidays; and making a choice among innumerable options add to the range of causes of stress.

Life events can be stressors, for example, birth of a child, abortion, illegitimate birth, elderly men and women caring for spouses who have been hospitalized for series illness,[7] death of a loved one, witnessing or learning of violence to loved ones, divorce, threat to your life or bodily integrity, physical injury or harm, exposure to the grotesque, learning of exposure to a noxious agent, causing death or severe harm to another, school examinations, dropping out of school, migration and immigration, aging, caring for an infirm or aging relative, brevity of life and pain, and the inescapability of death.

In modern society, stress often stems from doing things that are at odds with your feelings, sensing that you do not have enough time to do what you want, juggling family and work, and feeling stretched while working at high gear. Family members live in different places and no longer provide support as families did in the past. The uncertainty of the workplace—businesses closing and downsizing, mergers, reorganization, outsourcing, increased working hours, and technology's ability to keep employees tied to the job after business hours—creates stress. Central to the stress experience is an individual's sense of control.[8] Burnout at work as a result of a lack of personal control allowed in doing your job, lack of supportive work and family policies, tension with co-workers and overbearing bosses, insufficient lines of communication with management, and overwork cost American industry more than $300 billion in 2003. Stress reduces productivity, increases absenteeism, and escalates medical insurance and worker's compensation payments. Consider that the bill is in excess of ten times the cost of all strikes combined, or the total net profits of all the Fortune 500 companies. When a husband retires and his wife continues to work, usurping the traditional male role as the breadwinner leading an exciting life, stress is common.

The litany of stressors continues: Natural disasters such as the 2004 tsunami of unheard-of dimensions—nearly 150,000 people killed and villages and cities destroyed in at least eleven Asian countries—as well as storms, floods, tornados, hurricanes, earthquakes, fires, and life-threatening diseases such as cancer and AIDS; indeed, all illnesses and drug addictions are stressors. Hurricane Katrina, on August 28, 2005, caused the worst natural disaster in American history, destroying homes, neighborhoods, and lives over ninety thousand square miles. Even though there had been warnings, New Orleans was reduced to a sewage pit overnight as levees broke. Surging twelve-foot-deep waters catalyzed evacuation. Then came fires, bloated dead corpses decomposing in the streets for days, fetid waterborne disease, a decimated legal system of the New Orleans area, and the obliteration of courts and records and their support network, like no other disaster had caused before. This macabre scene and the ensuing relief fiasco in the richest and most powerful nation in the world revealed the federal government's ineptitude—after billions had been spent to make America safe from terrorism—and a racial and poverty divide. Other parts of Louisiana and coastal Mississippi and Alabama also suffered appalling devastation.

However, violence inflicted by human beings exacts a greater psychic toll than the impersonal cruelty of nature. For example, terrorists spread fear and panic in fragmenting contemporary society. Tel-Aviv University researcher Avital Laufer concluded from her survey of three thousand children ages thirteen to fifteen living in Israel and Jewish communities in the West Bank and Gaza that some 42 percent of Israeli children suffer from post-traumatic stress syndrome as a result of the wave of terror attacks that began in 2000. Seventy percent of these children said the terror attacks had had a "direct impact" on their lives.[9]

People with prior psychiatric conditions who had been improving frequently have setbacks. The impact of a distressing event is often exacerbated by other stresses, such as loss of jobs and displacement from homes. Caretakers and therapists are stressed to keep their own composure in confronting hair-raising incidents. There may be transmission of memory of violence from parent to children to grandchildren that shapes their inner and interpersonal and environmental worlds. A "victim" of victims hurt by calamities may have trouble coping with the inherent "radioactivity" of trauma.

## More Stress Today?

A *New York Times* front page headlined a series of articles on "The Stress Explosion."[10] Is stress greater today than it has been at other times? Probably not. But there is a greater awareness of stress, a concept that entered the medical literature in the early twentieth century. Soldiers experienced what was called shell shock in World War I, and combat fatigue in World War II. In 1954, concentration camp syndrome was recognized. Post-traumatic stress disorder was first conceptualized in 1980 with Vietnam War veterans who experienced three clusters of symptoms: intrusive thoughts about a traumatic event, emotional numbing and avoidance of a reminder of that event, and physiological hyperarousal.

Hardly a day passes when I don't read about stress in one area or another of our lives. We experience it, the news media report it, and medical researchers investigate it. Stress was a *Newsweek* cover story October 3, 2005. Three out of four Americans complain about chronic stress.[11] In the late 1980s, stress management programs began to make their way through society. Enthusiasts speak of a fifteen-billion-dollar industry. Vendors of stress relief sell books, videotapes, computer programs, vitamins, and cosmetics.

## Healing through Dance

Dance has become part of the stress relief effort, health promotion, and wellness programs. Among several techniques, such as body movement, roleplaying, and relaxation, that people use to cope with stress today, dance is widespread, engaging professionals, amateurs, viewers, and clients in dance therapy. Arthur Murray studios advertise their dance classes as a way to "relieve your stress" (WTOP radio, September 14, 2004). Extracurricular activities offered to university students include dance as an antidote to stress. Similarly belly dance/Middle East dance studios and women's self-help groups turn to dance as a stress reliever. Advertisements like "*Dance* away the blues—release that stress!" are common.

Business organizations sponsor stress reduction programs to cut staff absenteeism and boost productivity and morale. For example, the Johnson and Johnson Company learned that its wellness program paid for itself with a result of lower employee hospitalization costs and a 13 percent decrease in sick days.[12]

Denver's Initiative 101 on the electoral ballot requires the city to adopt "systematic stress-reducing techniques or programs." Jeff Packman, leader of the low-key campaign for the peacefulness plan, said, "I don't get too excited when people make fun of us. Sarcasm is what always greets innovation. You know, they laughed at Einstein. The fact is, stress builds up in a community the same way it does in a person. We know that there are remedies on the personal level...there are also proven, peer-reviewed scientific techniques that can reduce stress and tension on a community-wide level."[13]

Dance is taking on a bigger role in patient recovery. A growing number of leading medical institutions, including those associated with universities such as Johns Hopkins, Stanford, Dartmouth, and Vanderbilt. Georgetown University Hospital oncologist and professor of medicine Robert Warren supports the therapeutic use of the comfort and soothing aspect of the arts, which have the ability to remind patients that they are more than their illness.[14]

To prevent or respond to stress, some people talk with friends, drink, eat, become violent, or turn to religion. Yet other people dance—do it or watch it. Dance to heal? Yes. Dance to prevent stress? Yes. Can dance itself be a stressor? Yes, that too, for dancers, parents, choreographers, companies, production staff, dance critics, and others in the dance world. And as with all healing approaches, there are counterindications.

Is it unusual to resist, reduce, or escape stress through dance? All living organisms have methods of self-protection. Since early history and across cultures, humans have turned to dance, a full expression of mind and body

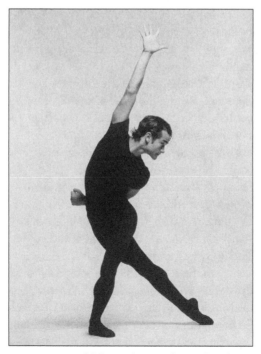

**Figure P.3.   Pressured (Photo of Rasta Thomas by Chris Dame)**

and self, as a talisman against stress. Many difficulties previously labeled in various ways from the time of our earliest records are now subsumed under the term *stress*. So, looking through history, one can assume that problems faced by a group caused many of its members to feel stress. Their dance response to deal with problems was in essence a way to deal with stress.

Although there are few statistically based and analyzed control studies that demonstrate specific relationships between dance and stress, compelling supportive case material and some stand-alone studies exist. Certainly an array of related studies that build upon each other over a five- to ten-year period would be welcome. *Dance/Movement Therapists in Action: A Working Guide to Research Options*, edited by Robyn Cruz and Cynthia R. Berrol, offers ways of conducting research on the therapeutic uses of dance. *Measuring Stress in Humans: A Practical Guide for Field Research*, by medical anthropologists Gillian Ice and G. D. James, will offer help to assess dance-stress connections.

As in any developing body of research, it is useful to look for consistent patterns of findings among various studies. The conclusion in *The Great Psychotherapy Debate: Models, Methods and Findings* is that a particular type of therapy accounts for only a small portion of the success or failure of a given patient's psychotherapy. What is critical are "nonspecific effects—the therapist's skills, the quality of the bond formed between therapist and patient, and the patient's own motivation to change."[15]

We know that stress is a complex phenomenon. It encompasses social organization and individual biographies as well as links to themes of agency, control, identity, and mediating factors. In the same way that many people accept our grandparents' hand-me-downs of age-old remedies, like chicken soup for a cold, many people also accept the intuitive belief in the efficacy of dance. Trial-and-error experiments occur.

Moreover, there is theoretical justification for the propositions about dance and stress. There are also scientifically documented bodily and mental processes involved in dancing that help us to understand the dynamics of how dance-stress relationships work. But most significantly, dance is a form of exercise. Researchers have found that regular exercise is a critical component of ways we can guard against the ravages of stress and be resilient to it. Exercise alters our mood and improves mental health.[16] Exercise blunts the stress response. David Nieman, professor of health and exercise science, explains: "Exercise appears to be useful because as the individual adapts to the increase in heart rate, blood pressure, and stress hormones experienced during exercise, the body is strengthened and conditioned to react more calmly when the same responses are brought on during mental stress."[17] Depression and anxiety disorders, including various phobias, panic attacks, and obsessive-compulsive behavior, have been shown to be reduced with exercise. "Physical activity is still the best stress-coping mechanism going," says psychologist John Forety, director of the Nutrition Clinic at Baylor College of Medicine in Houston.[18] Nearly every set of recommendations for stress management includes exercise as a therapy for mental health problems, a means of coping and managing stress, and a way of preventing its onset.

Researchers argue that exercise releases a copious quantity of the opiates beta-endorphins—magical, morphine-like brain chemicals. These natural narcotics produce feelings of calm, satisfaction, euphoria, the sensation known as the "runner's high," and greater tolerance for pain. Other researchers say endorphins that are synthesized within the brain can influence mood, but endorphins synthesized by the adrenal glands do not cross the blood-brain barriers, the molecules being too large to reach the brain and unlikely to influence mood or the perception of pain.[19] However, they contend that exercise, like meditation, blocks out the stress of a person's environment by distracting the individual and by physically removing the stress-producing effects of the environment. Exercise raises body temperature improving blood flow in the brain, relaxes the nervous system and muscles, and alters electrical patterns in the brain. This activity tends to have a tranquilizing effect on body and mind, offering escape temporarily from problems. William P. Morgan and John S. Raglin found that the difference between meditation and exercise is a persistence effect: twenty to thirty minutes for meditation versus more than three hours for exercise. People who suffer depression ruminate on negative thoughts, so distraction is useful. Intensive physical training can evoke analgesic effects.[20]

Another benefit of exercise is the prevention of the stress of a negative self-image if one is overweight. Exercise prevents the accumulation of body fat by building muscle which burns fat and calories for weight loss. Disco dancing, for example, burns about 468 calories per hour for men, 338 for women; and walking burns 288 and 208 calories, respectively. Exercise increases the basal metabolic rate, whereas dieting to lose weight leads the body to reset and decrease its metabolism. Exercise also dispels pent-up aggressive drives.

Fatigue makes one more vulnerable to stress. Exercise makes the heart a more efficient pump, so the muscles of a physically fit person more effectively extract oxygen from circulating blood and lessen the buildup of fatigue-inducing lactic acid. In addition, exercise helps regulate biorhythms that improve sleep and enhance energy level and vigor. Physical training leads to a protective stress hardiness for dancing and life's pressures.

Exercise helps ward off stressful diseases. It increases sensitivity to insulin, the hormone that clears the blood of excess sugar. Weight-bearing exercise increases the calcium content of bones, warding off osteoporosis and debilitating fractures later in life. Exercise keeps joints mobile. Exercise increases circulating levels of prolactin (a peptide, or short protein chain), which appear to provide protection against some forms of stress-induced stomach ulcers. However, too much of a good thing, like high-intensity exercise, can negate the benefits or even increase anxiety.

The exercise of sensory-motor processes leads to a child's brain development for mental and social functions. Exercise increases the ability of the brain to hold information transiently. Moreover, exercise feeds brain cells with a heartier supply of natural substances called neurotropins that enhance brain cell growth, acting like a fertilizer on nerve cells and slowing brain-cell death that comes with aging. Exercise and learning can contribute to neurogenesis, the replenishment of the supply of nerve cells in the hippocampus, the region of the brain most vulnerable to the wear and tear of distress. Neurogenesis may help form stress-induced memories that remind one of danger. Stress blocks neurogenesis.

Why dance rather than engage in other forms of exercise or passive approaches to handle stress? Dance seems to have special characteristics, namely, exercise with distinct physical dimensions, affective patterns, and nonverbal language-like communication, as I will point out in the next chapter. Indeed, to dance is to be human. Cave paintings and artifacts with images of dance document its antiquity. Later historical records attest to the persistence of dance into the contemporary era. Even when dance has been repressed or suppressed, it reappears like a phoenix.

Moreover, dance offers what prose writing or reading offer—creative cognitive patterning, story telling, social interaction, workout of mind and spirit, and a dimension of spontaneity and fantasy. Both the sensory and the symbolic are privileged in dance.

## Itinerary across Time and Space

This book does not offer a prescriptive program laying out specific 1-2-3 dance steps to deal with stress. Rather, I suggest the potential of a medium that humans have drawn upon throughout time and across geographical space as a key weapon in their arsenal against stress. I present an illustrative catalog of cases that suggest dance as a strategy. I also explain how dance can induce stress. Another group of cases portrays the role of dance in contemporary psychotherapy.

I must admit my bias in regard to ways that peoples have used dance to avoid and buffer stress. Since 1946 when a pediatrician prescribed dance for my flat feet, dance has helped me to develop strength to ward off the debilitating effects of stress as well as to reduce its impact. My feet didn't improve, but through dance I have experienced catharsis, tension dissipation, physical and psychological relaxation, relief from depression, and euphoria.

As the following pages will reveal, dance in its infinite variety is a multi-faceted phenomenon. To be sure, at times dance itself may trigger stress for the doer or viewer. Along our path toward understanding the value of dance in stress management, those interested in the phenomenon of dance per se may find answers to some of their questions.

At the outset, in chapter 1, I explain what I mean by the terms *stress* and *dance*, and in chapter 2, I describe three key relationships between dance and stress, types of stress management approaches, styles of intervention in stress, and dance genres associated with stress.

Part II (chapters 3 through 7) describes some of the palette of dance experience, forms, and practices that individuals and groups in the past and around the world have drawn upon to adapt creatively to the exigencies of survival. People dance in relation to gods, demons, plagues, pestilence, sexuality, and identity.

As an anthropologist, I take a cross-cultural perspective and present dance practices related to stress that come from cultures different in many ways from our own. Culture refers to the values, beliefs, attitudes, and learned behavior shared by a group and learned through communication. Individuals contribute to culture, which is a dynamic ever-changing phenomenon.

For several reasons, a cross-cultural perspective is valuable. First, I draw upon material relating to dance and stress from families, villages, and societies that seems, at first glance, to have little in common with what is found in modern society. Yet in our contemporary, pluralistic world, we find vestiges of these traditions in homes, streets, and neighborhoods. History provides an enlightening record of where we have been and where we are. Moreover, we find common underlying patterns as a result of diverse people's common humanity.

Second, a cross-cultural perspective helps us to increase our repertoire of the spectrum of possibilities from which we may choose. By examining the dance practices of other societies, we can gain new insights and apply, with modification, certain approaches to our own situations. Not only does one generation pass down a cultural heritage to the next, but individuals also learn from other groups. A comparative perspective is often a mind stretcher, prejudice dissolver, and taste widener. Even though our social organization, cultural artifacts, and general technology have changed significantly over the millennia, there is little evidence that the human species' psychobiological inheritance has so changed. We still refer to Plato, and doctors find curative medicinal practices of isolated exotic people worthy of "civilized" people's attention. What works for one member of the human species just may work, as is or in transformation, for another, irrespective of the contextual complexity.

Third, a cross-cultural perspective can prepare health practitioners to deal better with neglected or underserved diverse populations, while recognizing underlying similarities among all groups. During the 1968 joint conference of the Research Department of the Postgraduate Center for Mental Health, the Committee (now Congress) on Research in Dance, and the American Dance Therapy Association, a number of clinicians reported that they were unable to effectively reach clients who were not middle-class white Americans. I discovered time and again in my various field research studies that all people do not express themselves or interpret movement in the same way.

For example, in exploring school children's social life in a multicultural, socially and economically mixed elementary school, I asked boys and girls in grades two, four, and six how they can tell if a child feels different emotions.[21] Several clues identified the same emotion. In answer to "How can you tell if a child is angry?" several children focused on arm-hand action and physical contact: "Sometimes they slug you," said a sixth-grade boy. A second-grade youngster put it this way: "They balls his fist; they pushing." The appearance of the entire body was a clue for other children: a sixth-grade girl remarked, "Sometimes they puff up." The stomping of feet also indicated anger. Children said the face attracted attention: "They roll the eyes at you, get all hunched up"; "When a boy gets mad, his lip start sticking out." Occasionally an expression intended to be friendly was interpreted otherwise, which triggered a fight.

Fourth, a cross-cultural perspective may widen the understanding of how people constitute meaning in dance movement. Because there are styles within an art culture, avant-garde participants may perceive images in abstract dance presentations that audiences accustomed to more traditional forms of art miss. A case in point: at one of the dance concerts of contemporary performer and choreographer Douglas Dunn, a couple performed a duet. Spectators offered opposing views on whether or not the dancers conveyed feeling in the dance before the first intermission and how they felt in response to what happened on stage. Forty-six percent saw *no emotion*. People unfamiliar with or hostile toward abstract renderings described the movement as mechanical, stilted, robot-like, and computerized. "It made me feel like I was watching androids or mechanical mannequins," said a respondent. Yet other audience members perceived contrasting emotions, although they differed in their personal feelings in response to the same emotions. Forty percent of the respondents observed eroticism, a rather strong emotion. A male engineer perceived this feeling in the intertwining and rolling of the couple on the floor, and he said it made him feel "horny." Another person viewed the dancing as "X-rated." A male lawyer saw ecstasy as the dancers were "lying as if spent," and he felt "excited."[22]

Part III turns to contemporary Western society. Chapter 8 focuses on how choreographers, dancers, and audiences manage stress through the medium of theatrical stage performance. Chapter 9 examines stressors in pursuing a professional dance career. Amateur dancers, too, deal with stress, as chapter 10 illustrates. Dance in its therapeutic manifestations is the subject of chapter 11, which, as in part I, includes theoretical and empirical underpinnings from psychology and science. A discussion of dancing without injury and for managing stress appears in the finale.

This book's intended audience includes anyone interested in dance or health, and scholars and students in the arts, humanities, and education, and social, behavioral, and medical sciences. Because I have written the book with a broad readership in mind, specialists may find certain sections familiar or even elementary. I beg their patience; the familiar material, I hope, will offer a comfortable map before moving into foreign terrain. As a pioneer study, this work should catalyze further exploration.

~

## CHAPTER ONE

# Evolution's Gifts

## Stress?

From the beginning of antiquity, psychological responses to extreme trauma have been the source of intellectual curiosity. Verses were written in cuneiform about the city of Ur's exposure to raid, plunder, and slaughter around 2028 to 2004 b.c., when the Elamites from the east and the Sumerians from the west attacked and destroyed the city. Hamlet speaks of "suffering the slings and arrows of outrageous fortune." Africans refer to the anger of the gods and spirits. Many people anguish over the state of oppression imposed by their conquerors and rulers as well as questions of identity. Pestilence evokes wonder.

The word *stress*, a popular term, came into the medical literature in 1914, with the work of physiologist Walter Cannon. He explored the specific mechanisms of responses to stress, referring to the physical or emotional tension caused by factors that alter a person's existing equilibrium. In the 1930s, the research of pioneer endocrinologist Hans Selye on the physiological systems involved in stress gave the concept wide recognition. Researchers discovered a continuous dialogue between the nervous, immune, and endocrine systems. In this internal body language, messenger molecules called peptides respond to anything extraordinary that occurs in the body. A peptide can direct the flow of immune system cells called macrophages, raise or lower body temperature, or create feelings of pain, joy, or sadness.

Selye says stress is the result of any demand upon the body, either a mental or somatic demand for survival and the accomplishment of our goals.[1] Stress is a process that occurs when individuals have to cope with demands that require them to function above or below their habitual level of activity. A stressor indicates force that produces strain when a person is pushed to the outer limits of a particular capacity.

Bruce McEwen, a preeminent researcher with more than three decades's experience tracing the specific ways in which the brain organizes the body's glands and immune system to meet demands during stressful events, uses the terms "allostasis" or "allostatic load" for distress. The concept of homeostasis is that there is a single optimal level for any measure in the body, which can be reached through a local regulatory mechanism. Allostasis recognizes that regulation can occur in many ways, each with its own consequences. McEwen's excellent book, *The End of Stress as We Know It*, informs the following discussion and provides research references.[2] Stress is a natural and necessary means of empowerment to ensure our safety and survival. The stress response gives us the energy tools to respond quickly to sudden emergencies while staying mentally alert and physically prepared to meet a challenge. Moreover, researchers have found that moderate and low levels of exposure to stress, and occasional flare-ups in response to stress, appear to spur the release of special protective proteins that can arrest cell damage and thereby increase longevity.[3] The hormonal response to stress is linked to the heat-shock mechanism, a switch that activates the genes that produce the proteins responsible for the cell's quality. These heat-shock proteins include the molecular chaperone proteins that detect, repair, or dispose of other proteins that may be unsound.

**You Judge**

Of course, stress is a matter of interpretation and degree, and it is both subjective and objective, as well as positive and negative. Causes of stress are a matter of how you respond to changing and, more importantly, conflicting demands in your life. Speaking to the Brain Connection to Education Spring Conference in 2000, reknowned stress researcher Robert Sapolsky referred to stress "as stuff we make up in our heads . . . insofar as we are smart enough to have invented this stuff and stupid enough to occasionally fall for it, potentially we have the wisdom to keep it all in perspective so that we're not done in by it."[4] In fact, in response to the same stressor, some people develop stress-related diseases and others don't.

Stress-related conditions are psychomatic. The mind and body work together to lead to health or illness. Problems associated with stress result from the complex interaction between the demands of the outside world and the body's capacity to manage potential threats.[5] Influences on this capacity include diet, exercise, and sleep patterns.

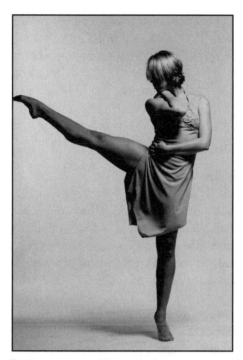

**Figure 1.1. Reflections on Stress (Photo of Adrienne Canterna by Chris Dame)**

It's not completely an issue of mind over matter, but McEwen reminds us that "the human mind is so powerful, the connections between perception and physiological response so strong, that we can set off the fight-or-flight response [discussed below] by just imagining ourselves in a threatening situation. This ability can be a source of power or an invitation to illness."[6] It is the brain's perception of stress that galvanizes bodily changes that are certainly real and increase your risk of getting diseases that make you ill. Moreover, repeated thoughts and actions can alter both the function and the structure of the neural networks in our brains.

Internal and external predispositions or immunizing factors modulate your response to stress. You may perceive stress without manifesting any objective, verifiable sign. Or, on the contrary, you may manifest stress and refuse to admit it, because admission would suggest self-weakness or inadequacy. Perception of stress depends on your personality within the context of your cultural and social groups. These shape your values about life events and structure social interactions with people who may become either stressors or supporters. Appraisal of events is relevant to your values, goals, and beliefs about yourself and the world. This variability means that you are what in common parlance is referred to as "cool," not easily perturbed. Or you are short tempered.

A situation that one culture deems stressful another may take in stride. Loud noise, for example, may be comforting or distressing, depending upon what people are used to. From infancy, the Inuit are accustomed to falling asleep easily in a noisy household. An outsider might find such a setting too stressful for a good night's sleep.[7] Competitive, hostile environments tend to create tensions that cooperative, friendly settings preclude.

**The Good and the Bad**
Stress may be beneficial, that is, be helpful in catalyzing adaptive, productive, and creative efforts to solve problems. Some people flourish under stress. Moderate amounts of discomfort are alerting and invigorating. You may undergo a stressful life event and suffer no immediate disability or permanent damage but realize psychological and social growth instead. The stressor might stimulate your commitment to achieving goals and induce healing processes.

Pursuing a passion for the glory of success and the potential for euphoria, some people deliberately seek out stress in such challenges as athletic competition or a dance career. Stress motivates these individuals to attain higher peaks of performance. Other people seek stress for therapeutic and religious reasons. Deliberately pushing the body and mind beyond normal limits through sensory overload to deprivation, as biological stress reactions cascade, may lead a person to experience euphoria, a vision, or mysticism.

There are other kinds of positive stress. Adrenaline, the hormone released during stress and anxiety, enhances memory.[8] Dance with a sensory overload may induce stress that in turn brings on a state of resistance or strength to reduce other stressors, that is, a cross-resistance, or provide a resilience to stress. During certain stress-inducing dances, participants may escape from the stresses of everyday toil for survival and achieve euphoria. An example of the stress paradox is that some executives thrive on stress. But a sluggish economy, widespread layoffs, and heightened scrutiny of business procedures raise the stress levels in many senior-level jobs.

Negative stress, or distress, occurs when the body's defenses against the harmful effects of stress become overworked and exhausted. Stressors are accompanied by specific side effects that include feelings of frustration and resentment, emotional outbursts, muscular tension, violence, withdrawal, depression (generalized feelings of hopelessness, despair, sadness, or pessimism), anxiety (foreboding about impending disaster), nervousness, trembling of the hands, rapid heartbeat, shortness of breath, increased perspiration, high blood pressure, difficulty in swallowing, headaches, diffuse aches and pains in the

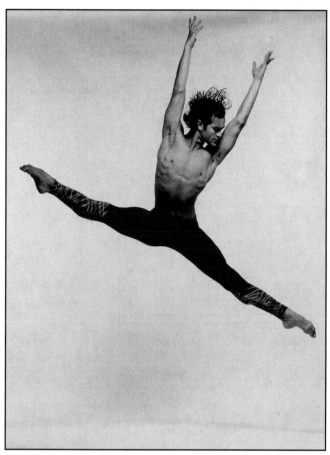

**Figure 1.2.  Challenge (Photo of Rasta Thomas by Chris Dame)**

joints, loss of appetite, fever, insomnia, skin eruptions, gastrointestinal disorder, thermal disturbances (icy hands despite heat, or hot body temperature in a cold environment), lowered resistance to disease, and problems of concentration (see figure 1.3).[9]

A host of serious mental and physical illnesses plague stress-ridden individuals. Doctors have estimated that emotional stress and its accompanying muscular tightness may contribute to about 80 percent of back problems. Agoraphobia (fear of being helpless in an embarassing or unescapable situation, and avoiding public places) and related panic attacks, thyroid disease, diabetes, asthma, heart disease, cancer, colitis, arteriosclerosis, sexual dysfunction, cessation of growth in children, gastric and duodenal ulcers, and sleep

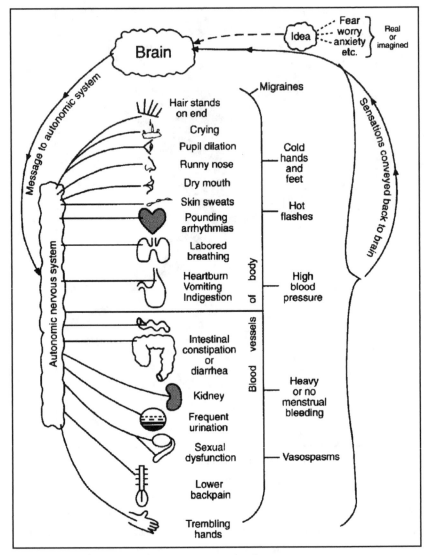

**Figure 1.3.  Impact of Stress**

deprivation are also maladies associated with stress. Periods of minor, chronic, or acute physical or psychological stress (including depression and shyness) suppress elements of the immune system that defend the body against invading microorganisms like viruses, bacteria, and toxins. Temperament affects the impact of stress and resistance to illness. Socially inhibited HIV-infected men have nearly eight times as many viral particles in their blood compared to

HIV-infected outgoing men.[10] Chronic distress is associated with brain damage, impaired memory and learning, and risk of Alzeimer's disease.[11] Shell shock in World War I, combat fatigue in World War II, concentration camp syndrome, and post-traumatic stress disorder are obviously distress. They shatter the meaningfulness of the self and the world. The extension of interest from military aspects of stress to its role in our routine daily existence during peacetime came about because modern war involved civilians sustaining the industrial machine. Stress became the umbrella for concepts like conflict, frustration, trauma, anomie, alienation, anxiety, and depression.

On one hand, what appears to be a maladaptive response may reduce social and psychological stress. On the other hand, what appears to be adaptive may be only the momentary escape during which an individual deals with the symptoms and not the causes of stress.

### Mobilizing for Fight or Flight

In what physiologist Walter Cannon called the *fight-or-flight* response, biological processes in the stress-response pattern automatically prepare the body for defense.[12] This, says Redford Williams, a stress researcher at Duke University Medical Center's Department of Psychiatry, "causes the hormones cortisol and adrenaline to be released, the sympathetic nervous system to fire off and the heart to pump four to five times more rapidly. Blood is shunted away from organs into muscles. When you are in this mode a good deal of the time your brain is scrambled, your thinking process doesn't work well, your judgment is clouded."[13]

Selye called the three phases of the stress-response pattern the *general adaptation*.[14] First, the body mobilizes to cope with irritation or harsh conditions in an *alarm reaction*. The body's defense during stress is to produce inflammatory hormones and then, in the second phase of the stress-response pattern, the stage of resistance, to produce from the adrenal cortex anti-inflammatory hormones that limit the extent of inflamation against stressors and return the body to normal. The balance and interaction of these defense responses affect the relative resistance of the body to harm during the stress process. If you continue to experience stress, the stage of exhaustion in which resistance declines develops. To survive stress, keep it short. Stress alters the body's immune system and places an extra burden on the heart and blood vessels. There is a "broken-heart syndrome." Emotional stress may precipitate cardiac events in people who are predisposed to such events.[15]

Brain power directs the process and production of the stress response. Emotion, a physiological change in response to an external stimulus, triggers a feeling (representation of that change in the brain). Feeling, or affect, is an indispensable accomplice in ensuring your survival and allowing you to think. A powerful emotion, such as fear, takes shape in the brain's amygdala, a structure adjacent to the hippocampus that is responsible for the emotional content of memory. Fright activates the amygdala, which in turn stimulates the stress hormone. This mechanism allows you to escape first and ask questions later.[16] A danger sign's pathway is from the eye to amygdala and then to the higher cortex and back to amygdala. If the message is a stick and not a snake, the cortex tries to abort the amygdala's alarm signals. But once an emotion is turned on, it is difficult for the cortex to turn it off. All extreme emotions cause the brain to trigger a physiological reaction. Brain cells called neurons fire electrical signals stimulated by seeing, hearing, or smelling and associated thoughts.

Psychologist Chris Brewin argues that traumatic memories are based on everyday mechanisms that respond in an unusual way.[17] This is because of the physiological effects of high levels of sustained arousal on the different brain structures involved in memory (the hypothalamic-pituitary-adrenal axis, prefrontal cortex, hippocampus, and amygdala). Brewin distinguishes two kinds of memory: the VAM (verbally accessible memory) system has information that has had more conscious processing, and the SAM (situationally accessible memory) system, a lower-level, image-based system containing more-detailed sensory information with less conscious processing. Another set of processes involved in response to trauma relates to the impact on the victim's beliefs and identity. The post-traumatic stress syndrome problem is in large part due to a person's memories involving extreme fear or horror.[18]

Healing, it is believed today, involves detailed repeated exposure to traumatic information and the modification of maladaptive beliefs about events, behavior, or symptoms. Brewin says that cues to retrieval of memory (e.g., the street in which a person was attacked, the color of a car that hit him or her) need to be associated with a sense of current safety. "Most kinds of trauma-related images can . . . be manipulated in the imagination to produce a different or more reassuring outcome."[19] He believes treatment first requires the abolition of flashbacks and nightmares, which can be brought about by having the patient focus on detailed sensory images of traumatic scenes and reencode information into the VAM system. This alternative memory in the presence of reminders of trauma competes with original memories in the SAM system to determine which one will be retrieved. The second part of treatment is to reestablish positive beliefs and identities and deactivate negative beliefs and feared identities that the trauma has evoked.

Scientists and mental health experts have found that merely the images on television, video, or the Internet, such as those of hostage taking (people, flanked by masked men carrying swords or AK-27s, begging for their lives), innocent people beheaded or otherwise executed, haunt and stress us in our role as secondary witnesses to the horrific acts of our time.[20] These images have embedded threats and fears into our memories, and they reemerge in debilitating ways. For primary and seconday trauma, dance therapy (see chapter 11) focuses on deactiving the paralyzing memories and promoting positive beliefs and identities.

The fight-or-flight syndrome does not require an emergency; indeed, everyday worries and pressures or the anticipation of a threatening situation or extraordinary excitement may trigger the response. Stress upsets the normal cycling of brain chemicals. The stress response begins in the forebrain, where a structure called the hypothalmus sends a message to the adrenal glands seated atop the kidneys. Answering, the adrenals spill out the stress hormone adrenaline and speed up the heart rate to deliver the adrenaline through the bloodstream to the major muscles that must be activated to fight or flee. Breathing accelerates to bring more oxygen as the bronchial tubes in the lungs dilate and extra oxygen reaches the brain to help keep us alert. The skin's blood vessels constrict—creating the sensation of hair standing on end—to preclude too much bleeding in the event of injury. Adrenaline also triggers a substance, fibrinogen, to speed up blood clotting.

Cytokines, proteins produced by immune cells, activate the second major phase of stress response. Through the hypothalmus, the brain produces an excess of the corticotropin-releasing hormone (CRH), which sets off a series of chain reactions throughout the body, giving it increased speed and strength. CRH stimulates the pituitary gland to produce molecules of adrenocorticotropic hormone (ACTH). This chemical excess moves into the bloodstream to stimulate the adrenals to overproduce cortisol, another chemical that induces the formation and/or release from the liver of glycogen, which can be converted into sugar in the bloodstream and thus provide more energy. The liver also burns protein for extra energy instead of converting it to muscle. At the same time, hormones mobilize fat reserves and release them into the bloodstream in the form of free fatty acids that the muscles can use as fuel.

Nerve fibers signal the adrenal gland to secrete the hormone epinephrine during fear, and norepinephrine during anger. These two hormones speed up the heart to increase blood pressure and pump extra blood to the muscles and brain. Pupils of the eyes widen as some blood vessels dilate. Other blood vessels supplying the stomach and intestine constrict inhibiting activity in these areas. In this way, the need for food is decreased, and the oxygen and blood supply to the brain and muscles for fighting or fleeing is increased.

Your immune system is a network of specialized cells and chemical messengers that allow you to survive in a hostile environment with viruses, bacteria, and other harmful foreign substances. The system communicates with the brain and the endocrine system and influences how you feel and behave. In

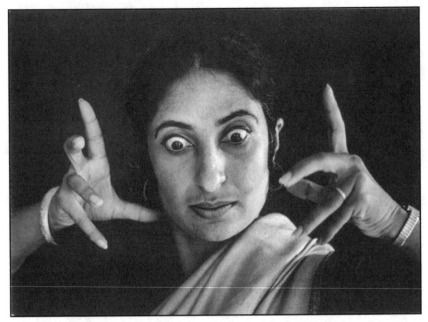

**Figure 1.4.** Anger (Photo of Nilimma Devi in Kuchipudi Dance. Courtesy of Sutradhar Archives)

turn, your behavior affects the immune system's work. In the stress response, the immune system's infection-fighting white blood cells rally to the blood vessel walls, prepared to reach whatever body part suffers injury. A temporary bulwark against infection also kicks in at a moment's notice to let you fight, stand firm, bolt to safety, or concentrate on the task at hand. The brain releases endorphins, natural painkillers, during a stress-response crisis. However, high levels of cortisol shut off production and action of cytokines that initiate the immune response. The immune system partially shuts down so that the body does not overreact and attack itself.

After the sympathetic system goes into action, the parasympathetic system begins to operate in order to conserve energy and allow the body to rest. Pupils constrict, blood pressure and heart rate lower, and digestive processes resume. The kidneys excrete excess cortisol, epinephrine, and norepinephrine into the urine.

### Too Much of a Good Thing: Damage
Interestingly, only the human animal can keep the hypothalamic-pituitary-adrenal axis going indefinitely because of how our faculties of perception,

thought, and emotion are produced in the brain and connected to the stress response. Memories that help you remember aspects of your daily life lie in the hippocampus, which also stores memories with strong emotional content, as it engages with the adjacent amygdala. A powerful emotion sears a memory into the brain's structures.

The paradox of the beneficial, powerful, and sophisticated fight-and-flight defense response is that it can become lethal. Envision a downpour that fertilizes the crops versus a flood that devastates them. Relentless stress—chronic stress, or distress—is a dangerous biological minefield that causes endocrine and autonomic changes that can alter the immune system's operation. Overproduction of cortisol can harm the hippocampus, which registers events and the context in which they occur and helps turn off the stress response after the threat has subsided. High levels of cortisol can shrink nerve cells in the hippocampus and halt the creation of new hippocampal neurons—changes also associated with aging and memory problems. When cortisol remains chronically elevated, it acts with insulin levels to send fat into storage at the waist.

Normally protective mechanisms become overburdened as a finely tuned feedback system is overcharged and runs amok causing damage. Numerous studies demonstrate the links between chronic stress and poor health.[21] The immune system ceases to function through the destruction of white blood cells or suppression of their activity. Even the body's immune organs may atrophy. Susceptibility to infections and disease—cardiovascular problems, colds, allergies, asthma, diabetes, colitis, chronic fatigue syndrome, fibromyalgia, eczema, and ulcers—follows. Stress can exacerbate disease.[22] If stress reactions become habitual, muscles and tendons shorten and thicken and connective tissue is deposited, causing a general consolidation of tissues. Cognitive function is impaired. Women are likely to experience dysmenorrhea, defined as menstrual pain for two or more days, when they experience high levels of stress.[23] Stress may turn a person's hair gray abruptly; researchers have investigated how stress gets "under the skin" and found psychological stress speeds up the aging of the body's cells at the genetic level.[24] The distress that causes clinical depression or anxiety can even cause parts of the brain to atrophy.

When you neither fight nor flee because physical action in the immediate situation is inappropriate, biochemical elements of energy may remain in the body. For example, fats released that are not metabolized may be deposited in the internal lining of the arteries. A repetition of such patterns of enduring stress may lead to atherosclerosis, an obstruction narrowing the arteries. This is one of several stress-related problems that contribute to cardiovascular diseases. Consequently, the mobilization capacity is likely to be maladaptive if you do not use the energy generated. It can be released in physical exercise, including dance, varieties of which I will describe in this book. Dance is a means to resist and reduce stress as well as achieve euphoria through its emotional, feeling, physical, and cognitive characteristics.

## Humans Dance

It is appropriate to point out the components of dance that make it a good medium for dissipating stress as well as to prevent it and escape it. Contrary to what many people think, dance has not only physical and emotional elements but cognitive ones also. So what is dance?

Considering the views of various groups worldwide, my observations of many dance forms, and a survey of the literature on behavior generally called dance, I think dance can be most usefully conceptualized in the following way: human behavior composed (from the dancer's perspective, which is usually shared by other members of the dancer's culture) of purposeful, intentionally rhythmical, and culturally patterned sequences of nonverbal body movements other than ordinary motor activities. The motion (in time, in space, and with dynamics) has inherent and aesthetic value. Aesthetics, in a cross-cultural perspective, refers to notions of appropriateness and competency held by the dancer's cultural group. And a group's dances, such as ballet and hip-hop, may have different aesthetics. Of importance to dealing with stress is the fact that dance has the potential to transform the dancer and onlooker. Elsewhere I have discussed the impact of dance for the individual and society at great length.[25]

### Body Motion and Feeling

In dance, the human body instrument releases energy through muscular responses to stimuli received and sent by the brain. This instrument may contract and release, flex and extend, gesture, and move from one place to another. The physical activity of dance is multisensory, engaging the sight of performers moving in time and space, the sounds of physical movements, the odors of physical exertion, the feeling of kinesthetic activity or empathy, and the sensations of contact with other bodies or the dancer's environment.

Dance may increase your energy and provide a feeling of invigoration. As regular aerobic exercise, dance makes the body work more, demand more oxygen, and use it more efficiently.[26] When the body uses oxygen efficiently, it requires less oxygen for a given amount of work. Aerobic capacity depends on the ability to rapidly breathe large amounts of air (efficient lungs), forcefully deliver large volumes of blood (powerful heart), and effectively deliver oxygen to all parts of the body (effective vascular system).

The exercise of dance increases the circulation of blood carrying oxygen to the muscles and the brain and alters the level of certain brain chemicals, as in the stress-response pattern. Vigorous dancing induces the release of endorphins thought to produce analgesia, euphoria, and feelings of transcendence similar to the runner's high. The change in oxygen distribution to the brain and blood-sugar levels affects how you feel. Maintaining a blood-glucose level within certain limits is critical for the body (the brain consumes a major portion of glucose, roughly a fifth of the body's calories, at rest). Normal hormonal regulation helps maintain the blood-glucose level. Beta cells in the pancreas constantly monitor blood-sugar levels and release the hormone insulin, the "fuel coordinator," accordingly.[27] However, without food or in cases of prolonged dancing, a performer becomes stressed: glucose supplies in circulation begin to dwindle, and low levels of insulin initiate the mobilization of stored fuels in the muscles. Because the muscles cannot convert glycogen into glucose for release into the blood, the muscle-carbohydrate stores in one area are of little use for muscles elsewhere in the body. The liver acts as the major energy transformer and produces and releases glucose into the bloodstream by breaking down its stores and increasing the uptake of raw materials to produce glucose. If liver-glycogen stores are depleted from prolonged dancing or low carbohydrate intake, and depleted fat stores restrict the availability of free fatty acids for energy needs due to poor nutrition, the liver may not be able to meet the demands of a situation, and hypoglycemia may set in. Symptoms include sweating, fatigue, spasms, numbness, and heart palpitations.

Energetic dancing, high-speed effort, sensory rhythmic stimulation in more than one sensory mode (kinetic and sonic action through musical accompaniment), and low-key dancing over long periods of time may also change your brain-wave frequencies and amount of adrenalin. These changes induce giddiness or other altered states of consciousness (the feeling of a qualitative shift in thinking, disturbance in sense of time, loss of control, change in body image, perceptual distortion, change in meaning, sense of the ineffable, feelings of rejuvenation, and hypersuggestibility).

The accumulation of by-products of muscular exertion in the blood results in fatigue and an oxygen debt (the inability of the body to take in as much oxygen as is being consumed by the muscular work). Sometimes dancers hyperventilate, or overbreathe. When you are anxious or excited, you breathe faster than normal. Consequently, you exhale more carbon dioxide, which changes the body's chemical balance. This change alters blood flow, the amount of circulating oxygen, and the way nerves and muscles work, leading to faintness, dizziness, and lightheadedness.

Significant psychological benefits of physical exercise for persons with clinically diagnosed anxiety disorder have been questioned. The issue is that intensive muscular exertion can have symptoms associated with panic attacks, namely, rapid heart action, palpitations, shortness of breath, and sweating, and might precipitate or elevate an attack. However, researchers have found that exercise does not precipate or elevate an attack; patients can learn to expect and recognize similar symptoms during exercise.[28]

The physical exercise of dance may be an end in itself, the purpose being the pleasure of doing. Or dance may be part of courtship, mating, the promotion of solidarity and cooperation, religious or spiritual expression, preparation for work or war (as in many non-Western societies in which dance serves as military training)—and healing. Dance serves a wide spectrum of purposes, often several simultaneously, including preventing and coping with stress that may even be outside a person's awareness.

Because dance is different in some ways from other aspects of daily life, its performance usually provides a change-of-life space that differs from the workplace, although there are work dances. In an atmosphere unlike the work environment, the dancer and onlooker may find a refuge for relaxation and kinetic thought (some expression is easier in dance than in verbal communication).

Dance may cause emotional changes and altered states of consciousness, flow,[29] and secular and religious ecstasy. These changes are often stress related. Flow is a feeling of creative accomplishment and heightened functions that is important in resisting, reducing, and escaping stress. Elements of flow include a centering of attention, loss of self-consciousness, sense of control, and the joy of taking action. Erik Bruhn, who for over thirty years presented the distillation of pure classical ballet, said he reached the height of euphoria four or five times in his career. "There have been certain moments on the stage where I suddenly had a feeling of completeness ... I felt like a total being. ... It was a feeling of I am. At those moments I had the sense of being universal ... but not in any specific form."[30]

Dances in communal settings often build up a spirit of elation that is infectious among individual dancers and spectators. The body is the first form of human power. Groups of people dancing together create a still more-powerful body. Enveloping closely together in group performance may be ecstatic, a "communal sneeze" (catharsis, which I will discuss later), escape to a dreamworld, or a supportive setting in which an individual copes with stress. However, note that the condition existing for one person in a group may be completely opposite to that of another.

The presence of social support has been found to decrease stress and to suppress salivary-free cortisol levels. An underlying biological mechanism for protection against stress is the neuropeptide oxytocin, which is present in the central nervous control of neuroendocrine responses to stress.[31] People with the combination of oxytocin and social support exhibited the lowest cortisol concentrations as well as an increased calmness and decreased anxiety.[32] In dance the social support of touching and being touched by others evokes a sense of well-being. The pleasant stimulus of touch triggers the release of the hormone oxytocin, which creates a psychological bond that appears to ward off some of the physical as well as psychological ill effects of stress.[33] Oxytocin also lowers blood pressure, heart rate, and cortisol levels for up to several weeks.[34] Moreover, oxytocin is a hormone associated with emotional safety.

Religious ecstasy involves a sense of shifting boundaries of time and consciousness, usually as a person passes from the secular realm to the sacred. Some cultures require temporarily changed eating or sexual patterns preceding dances, such as rites of initiation or healing rituals, to further heighten an altered state of consciousness or religious revelation.

## Body Language

We know that the sensuous aspects of the dance experience do not exist apart from any mediation of ideas. Drawing upon the same cortical faculties of the brain that operate in verbalization, dancers makes decisions about using their bodies in a particular way to send and receive messages to other dancers and spectators. The cognitive dimensions of dance may also arouse emotions and contribute to altered states of consciousness, flow, and religious exaltation.

Dance, like spoken or written language, communicates. We may think of dance as a text in motion, a visualization and embodiment of thoughts and feelings expressed directly or symbolically. Your thinking, through words or dance, about concepts, events, and feelings may be emotional. In addition to being an outlet for physical and emotional energy, dance has communicative potential that is especially relevant to trauma victims. Dance can often express what words cannot, and multisensory communication packs more of a wallop in persuasion than mere words are able to. Modern-dance genius Martha Graham put it this way: "To me, the body says what words cannot.... Dancing is very like poetry. It's like the poetic lyricism sometimes, it's like the rawness of dramatic poetry, it's like the terror—or it can be a terrible revelation of meaning."[35]

Dance is a venue for storytelling and "talking it out," a commonly accepted form of therapy. Giving voice to grief is frequently part of healing. The nonverbal "speech" used in dance can provide a narrative or poetic means of learning to cope with stress, to understand it and your feelings, and then to go on more satisfactorily with your life. Dancing is active and volitional control. The need to focus on the dance elements of time, space, effort, and relating to others in space is empowering. Movement is both a metaphor and an actualization of change that alters the habitual way you use your body.[36] Because of widely held misperceptions about dance, it is important to distinguish the dance of humans from the dancelike movements of other animals or the spontaneous emotional kinetic expression of children. As humans evolved, the programmed action sequences (developmental instinctual behavior) characteristic of other animals tended to be replaced by actions in which cultural learning and individual purpose played a greater role. Consequently, in contrast with other animals and young children, more-mature humans select action patterns. The basis for this contrast lies in the evolution of the human brain. It expanded in size and became restructured in the cerebral cortex to permit greater memory storage and multiple means of fine perceptual discrimination, coordination, integration, and novel classification. Human evolution also led to increased dependency and socialization of offspring. These changes allow the transmission of a cultural heritage, which includes nonverbal communication. And within this domain lies dance. Notwithstanding individual creativity, a dancer's performance reflects a cultural heritage.

Following cultural rules, humans in their dances can voluntarily express or withhold emotions and ideas distanced in time and space from immediate stimuli. Using their bodies, dancers can choose rhythms with which to harmonize or counter. Their nonverbal movements are other than ordinary motor activities. A dance walk is not, for example, merely a means to move from one place to another but also a way to fulfill aesthetic values.

Through dance, humans have the capacity to communicate abstract concepts, to project experience beyond their own, to alter feeling and thought, and to transform them symbolically through various patterns. Such transformation occurs through different devices and spheres for sending messages, as I will point out later. The linguistic analogy may be helpful here. Dance is often less like prose than it is like poetry, with its suggestive imagery, rhythm, ambiguity, nuances recognized over time, multiple meanings, and latitude in form. In a dance performance, as in spoken and written languages, we may not see the underlying universal and cultural structures and processes, but merely their evidence. Structures are a kind of generative grammar—a set of rules specifying the manner in which movements can be meaningfully combined. Semantics refers to the meaning of movement, whether it is the style itself or some reference beyond the movement.

As in language (with its words, sentences, and paragraphs), dance has a movement vocabulary composed of steps and phrases that may comprise realistic or abstract symbols and evoke an affective mood. It is important to note that dance can be symbolic even when a dancer intends no such communication. From their own exprience, spectators are able to find associations in the visual images dancers frame for scrutiny and to inscribe meaning. The dancer's body is a "natural" symbol. Societies at times of stress symbolically shroud the boundaries of the body with rituals, including dance, to preserve it.[37]

Dancers are social commentators. Their performance may mirror what is in life, either as a validation or as a critique. Alternatively, dance may suggest what might be, through reversing usual actions, mocking the status quo, or presenting innovation. Whichever way, social dominance patterns in the broader society usually appear in the production of dance as well as the images of performance. Assuming an intent of communication, what contributes to received messages in the performer-audience exchange? It appears that shared knowledge and expectations are critical to getting an intended message. Understanding may vary according to the spectator's knowledge about dance, whether the spectator is an outsider to a society, a knowledgeable observer, or an insider (including a dance expert such as a critic, guru, movement analyst, dance teacher, choreographer, a dancer as executor of movement, or a dancer as creative interpreter of movement).

The importance of dance in communication lies in the fact that there are alternative ways of knowing and of glossing experience, and different types of communicative competencies, including bodily kinesthetic competence.[38] Some people are imagers. Furthermore, individuals do not possess a single conscious mechanism that is privy to the sources of all their perceptions and actions.

## Afterword

Both stress and dance are multifaceted and involve mind, body, and potential, interpretation and action. Stress and dance are subjective and objective as well as positive and negative. We have seen that what is stress to you may not be so to another person. There is good and bad stress. We have the evolutionary gift of being able to muster up defenses for self-defense. But too much of the stress-response mobilization can cause much harm. Through its physical energy and cognitive direction, dance is a means to resist, reduce, and escape stress. Now that we have set the stage by introducing some of the complexities of stress and of dance in general, let us turn to more specific kinds of relationships between them.

~

## CHAPTER TWO

# Dance-Stress Coupling

## Intentions and Consequences

Dance can have consequences that are intended and recognized by the participants, and those that are not. For example, a group may consider a dance celebrating the birth of a child to encourage the group's fertility, but the contribution of the dance to group solidarity or an individual's release of tension may not be recognized. You can deduce some meaning of a dance from the social and cultural settings as well as from theoretical concerns beyond the experience one culture alone provides. One or more psychological processes may be involved in the dance-stress phenomenon.

There is a difference between the dancer and viewer. The dancer creates, performs, and feels the dance, whereas the viewer may have empathy and vicarious experience. Performers often "speak" for their audience, indeed, their community, especially in ritual settings. Dancers may also be viewers when they perform before a mirror, see each other moving in a group, or see themselves on film or video. Note that people learn to dance in different ways: by watching, being coached, and taking classes or participating in therapy (see chapters 2, 9, 10, and 11).

Preventive, remedial, and inducive dance-stress connections are not mutually exclusive. Some dances are prophylactic and may also be performed in a crisis situation to reduce, escape from, or eliminate stress. Yet the same dances may, for some individuals under specific conditions, induce stress. The reason a dance may induce stress for one person or group and for another person or group resist or reduce stress is related to the person or group's views about the body and dance, personality, situation of time and place, and pervading cultural and social contexts.

It is important to point out when discussing the power of dance that it is usually not the dance alone that can effect changes. Who does what, when, where, how, with and to whom, beliefs, and the accoutrements of dance, such as music, costume, and sometimes incense and drugs, contribute to the efficacy of dance to assist people to resist, reduce, or escape stress.

## Music

Music plays a special role in most dance. Although there are exceptions, it is music that drives the dance movement. Relevant to the dance-stress connection, music contributes to the emotions and feelings of performers and observers. Sounds can physically bombard or soothe people and evoke associations. Music and dance may be intertwined on an equal status, or one may be dependent upon the other. Dance may be an adjunct of music or vice versa. There may be mirroring, opposition, and interweaving. Musicians may play instruments and also dance. In many African groups and in flamenco, musicians interact with the dancer, each giving the other clues as to what should transpire. Sometimes the dancer's rhythmic pattern follows the musicians'. At times the dancer contributes a distinct rhythm as part of the orchestral whole. Music visualization is a common pattern by which dancers interpret music.

## Dance: A Stress Vaccine

Dance may be a kind of stress innoculation. Through its interconnected cognitive, physical, and affective powers, dance may develop a person's enhanced well-being and greater tolerance to stressors.

### The Mind Matters
Using the imagery of kinetic discourse, dance may recount anticipated events that have potential anxiety or feared consequences. Presenting these embodied concepts or narratives may enable individuals to play with them, to distance them, and consequently to make them less threatening. This action is like a rehearsal. Failure is also acceptable and benign, because dance, after all, is only play and lacks the impact of real-life failure. If you don't like a performance scenario, you can create another. Past and current experiences may also be enacted through dance. These expressions have the potential to move an individual to evaluate problems, consider resolutions, and act in a constructive way outside the dance setting.

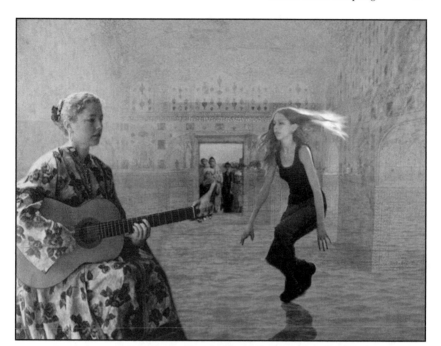

**Figure 2.1. Playing on Water in an Andalusian Palace (Artwork of Julia Banzi, guitar, and Zahra Banzi, dance, by Tarik Banzi, www.andalus.com)**

The effect of a dance activity depends in part upon the meaning a participant attributes to it. Dance may give an individual a sense of self-mastery through being in charge of the body and its actions, physical health, and appearance. The sense of self-mastery contributes to a positive self-perception, body image, and self-esteem—perceptions that help an individual resist stress.

Religious *beliefs* determine *possession* and *trance* states achieved through dancing that causes an excitation of vestibular apparatus and an altered state of consciousness with symptoms of dizziness, spatial disorientation, hallucinations, and muscular spasms. Trance is a sleeplike state characterized by reduced sensitivity to stimuli and the loss or alteration of knowledge of what is transpiring. Contact with supernatural entities through possession and trance provides guidance for individuals and their communities.

Before the birth of Jesus, Plato argued in *The Republic* that the soul or spirit benefits from regular vigorous activity. Effects of such exercise movement have been mentioned as beneficial by philosophers from the time of Plato and Aristotle.[1] Some contemporary dancers find dance a spiritual experience and a way to bliss. For example, Gabrielle Roth explains: "I feel my soul in my body when I dance . . . I believe we each hold a spark of the original light of creation within us. I've seen it light up people's faces and bodies when they dance. In a thousand ways it has been revealed to me that God is the dance and we need only to disappear in the dance to liberate the sexual, cretive, and sacred aspects of the soul."[2]

**Physical Immunization**
The contribution of dance to physical fitness may immunize an individual against the negative effects of stress. Exercise reduces the risk of certain stressful life-threatening diseases. A Harvard University alumni study showed that moderate exercise can help prevent heart attacks and lower blood pressure and total serum cholesterol while increasing the levels of the protective cholesterol-carrying high-density lipoprotein (HDL).[3] Physically active women are less likely than sedentary women to develop breast cancer. Exercise also helps to ward off adult-onset diabetes, strokes, depression, and other illnesses mentioned in chapter 1.

Dancing conditions the individual to be able to reduce, eliminate, or avoid chronic fatigue or lessen the impact of acute fatigue, both of which are symptoms of stress. A sense of invigoration is experienced through the increased flow of oxygen delivered to the brain and other body tissues. Some dances have aerobic patterns, movements that stimulate heart and lung activity for a sufficiently long period to produce behavioral changes in the body.

Dance may prevent the stress of premenstrual discomfort. Some women experience one or more emotional, physical, or behavioral symptoms (irritability, anxiety, fatigue, depression, bloating and weight gain, breast tenderness, headache, cravings for particular foods, and insomnia) during the week or two prior to menstruation.

Maintaining or achieving an optimal level of physical fitness through dance can contribute to the overall quality of the later years of an individual's life. Aging is a form of stress in the sense of the individual's loss of ability to adapt to the environment. There is a decline in elasticity of the major blood vessels; increase in resting pulse and blood pressure; degeneration of cardiac structures; loss of muscular and skeletal strength; decreased flexibility of joints comprised of cartilage, ligaments, tendons, and synovial fluid; slower reaction time; reduced ability to think clearly; and greater susceptibility to depression. Aging of individuals in cultures with limited expectations and roles for the elderly is often accompanied by melancholy, crankiness, and loss of satisfaction with one's looks. Dancing ameliorates some of the stressful effects of aging—decline in mental functioning and physical discomfort—through building fitness and endurance.[4] Dance builds coordination, agility, and muscular strength in the limbs and torso. Moreover, dance helps prevent osteoporosis, a disorder in which bones lose calcium and become brittle. This disorder causes more than one million spontaneous fractures a year in people over forty-five years of age, especially postmenopausal women. Like any other body tissue, when bone is stressed it hypertropies, when unstressed it atrophies.[5] Dancing in couples or groups involves touch and requires attention to both partners and steps, all of which are cognitively stimulating.

Most intriguing is a report that links dance to the association of chronic distress with brain damage, impaired memory and learning, and risk of Alzeimer's disease.[6] Neurologist Joe Verghese's team has studied what activities "stretched" minds and lowered the risk of seniors developing Alzheimer's disease.[7] Those who did crossword puzzles cut the risk by 38 percent; those who played instruments, 69 percent; those who played board games, 74 percent; and those who danced lowered the risk by 76 percent. Physical activities like group exercise and team games had no significant impact on warding off the onset of Alzheimer's. However, ballroom dancing has the mental demands of remembering dance steps and executing them in response to music, and coordination with a partner or group in space without bumping into other dancers. Certainly, dance helps to resist and reduce stress by decreasing the possibility of having a debilitating disease.

Inherent in the exercise of dance and its resulting prevention of injury, physical disability, or psychological tensions (emanating from, for example, confronting sensitive themes in dance or experiencing stage fright, as described in chapters 8 and 9) is a natural tranquilizing effect. This may improve a dancer's problem-solving capability.

## Dance: A Stress Buster

Dance is a remediative intervention to cope with stress. Dance's ability to help an individual cope with stress often functions in the same way that it does to help prevent stress. For example, dance may discharge repressed aggression, dissipate anxiety, provide a sense of mastery that causes a corresponding change in self-perception and self-esteem, and induce possession and trance. However, dance as a psychological treatment is similar to other treatments that work well for some people who have specific problems under particular conditions.

As a way to dissipate stress, dance has at least three manifestations: confrontation with stressors to reduce stress, diversion from stress, and relaxation of stress-induced muscle tension. All three patterns to cope with stress may involve catharsis as well as other psychological processes. *Catharsis* (also known as abreaction) in dance is a complex physical-cognitive-affective process of recollecting and releasing repressed emotions and tensions and thereby coming to terms with them. The process encompasses feeling anxiety or conflict and then releasing energy and frustration, and discharging distressful emotions in a substitution for action against the source of the problem.[8] Insight—understanding and evaluating one's own mental functioning (including recognizing the irrationality of some of one's impulses) to bring about psychological change—is often a concomitant of catharsis.

## Confronting Stressors

Many people in the United States have developed a dislike for the stresses of modern society characterized by the technological postindustrial revolution of mechanization and impersonality. Some of these individuals confront such stressors by turning to dance. They perceive dance as a pristine human-sentient phenomenon, a basic form of expression and communication, and an ennobling way of thinking, feeling, and moving that is under the individual's own control.

Because the nondance arts in the mid-twentieth century centered on form and abstraction (with the human body appearing, if at all, as disembodied and rootless), dance may have come into its own, in part, to meet the need for the aesthetic presence of the whole human body, self-exploration, and self-definition. The "lived-in body," even when presented in "abstract" formalist dance, symbolically sustains the individual's power in our mechanized society.[9] Through dance training and practice, you marshal power to discipline the instinctive and culturally patterned movements of the body. As a result, dance achievement shows control over the body and freedom to use it in a particular way, dominance, and ascendance comparable to the human conflict in bullfighting. This sense of mastery attracts some people to the dance profession. Consistent with the Enlightenment ideal that the arts should be instruments in controlling nature, dancers shape the rhythms of life and make the difficult look simple in testament to human competency and potential. Moreover, control through dance can relieve the stress of a poor self-image from obesity.

Healthy people coping with stress and those with stress-induced mental illness[10] need ways to communicate as a major redressive tool. Consequently, Western dance therapy, discussed in chapter 11, helps a client by focusing on the individual as well as the person's past and present close interpersonal relationships. In many cultures, dance responses to deal with stress convey messages to a stressed person's family and community and involve them in the production and performance.

Finding meaning through the use of storytelling is critical to coping with stress. By projecting their stories in the dance, individuals may be "working through" their difficulties. In this process, often under the guidance of a healer, either a shaman, a deity in the guise of a possessed dancer, or a Western-dance therapist, an individual faces the same conflicts until she or he is able to independently face and master these challenges in everyday life. Distancing or holding up a problem to scrutiny allows evaluation and possible resolution. The dance is potentially a creative way of dealing with conflict, learning about the self, and gaining insight.

Thomas Adeoye Lambo, an African psychiatrist, described some dancing, and its rhythm, vigorous movements, and their coordination and synchronization, as inducing some degree of catharsis.[11] The Greeks, too, spoke of dance and catharsis, a concept used in psychoanalysis to refer to the first step in understanding and eliminating underlying conflict. The year 1986 witnessed televised scenes of South African urban blacks dancing their protest against apartheid and white domination.

Nearly everywhere, dance, especially for recreation (ostensibly the most common kind of dance), may be cathartic. A pleasurable expenditure of energy, it is movement differing from everyday behavior and its associated pressures. Rapid turning leads to vertigo, to release, and to altered states of consciousness, which may clear the mind of distractions and bring about insight into one's self and community.

Humor is increasingly used as a way of dealing with stress.[12] Dance combined with humor packs a double whammy. With its power to increase the intensity of dancers' or spectators' emotions, music can enhance humor in dance. Laughter relaxes us, eases tension, and diverts attention from the unpleasant. Psychiatrist William Fry claims that laughing one hundred times a day is equivalent to ten minutes of strenuous rowing. Laughing strengthens the heart muscle. During a laugh, the throat sends blasts of air out of the mouth at seventy miles an hour from uncoordinated spasms in the throat and clears mucus from the lungs. The body pumps adrenaline, the heart rate increases, the brain releases the natural painkillers of endorphins and enkephalins, the lungs expel carbon dioxide, and muscles relax. Through laughter, some people cough out the wreckage of their past or find diversion from the unpleasant.

The Sidis, descendants of African slaves, sailors, servants, and merchants who sailed across the Indian Ocean to the west coast of India between the twelfth and late nineteenth centuries, illustrate the humorous dance-stress connection. In this case, the humor has sacred meaning and is in a sacred context. Ethnomusicologist Amy Catlin has found that the only remnant of their African culture is their music and dance, called *goma*.[13] It helps the Sidis cope with life, including their poverty. Sidis perform joyful and exuberant Sufi devotional music and dance, satirical praise dances to their saint, who is said to have given them the joy they express in their dances. Men dance with bent-knee

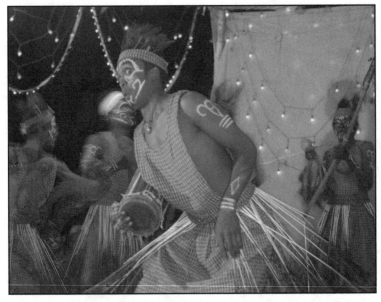

Figure 2.2.   Sacred Humor (Photo of Abdul Hamid Sidi, African-Indian Sufi dancer per-forming with Sidi Goma group at the urs—Festival of Saint—of Bhikan Shah Wali, Sachin, Gujarat, India, December 2001. Copyright by Nazir Ali Jairazbhoy,)

monkey walks and direct cheeky comical gazes at spectators. Intoxicating drum patterns that "speak" the *zikr* (danced) rhythmic prayers support the dancers, who perform virtuosic feats of agility and strength, gradually reaching an ecstatic climax. While the music gradually gets more rapid and excited, the dances unfold with constantly evolving individual and small-group acts of animal imitations. Catlin told me, "The essence of Sidi resistance, reduction, and escape through dance and otherwise is often based on humor (*mazaa*—also "enjoyment"), definitely a stress-relieving and vitalizing palliative—many outsiders who have seen their dances have commented on this effect."[14]

### Diversion from Stress

Besides portraying a problem in dance in order to manage it, another way of responding to stress is trying to avoid, escape, or transcend stress through vigorous or unending dancing that can, for physiological and psychological reasons already mentioned, lead to an altered state of consciousness, flow, catharsis, and euphoria. Dance, like other forms of intensive physical activity, often provides a healthy physical fatigue or distraction, which may abate a temporary rage crisis and thus allow "more enduring personality patterns to regain ascendancy."[15]

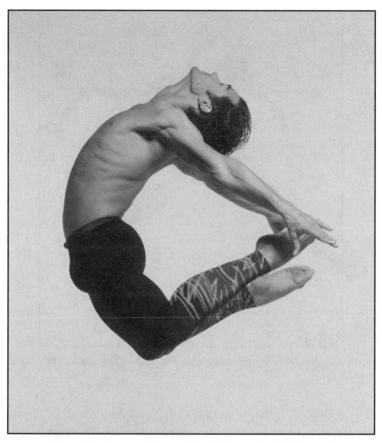

**Figure 2.3.   Escape (Photo of Rasta Thomas by Chris Dame)**

Many societies recognize the empirically supported supposition that physical exercise can alter psychological states. The contagious affect among dancers, musicians, and observers enhances distraction from stress. Like many people, I have experienced elation through dancing, both when I was in a good mood and when I was depressed or emotionally upset from a failure or misfortune. I had the sensation of soaring, being on a high (similar to the euphoria from ingesting alcohol or LSD) having light limbs, and feeling energy and power.

Enveloping yourself in dancing may provide a "time out" from anxious thoughts. The rhythmic motions of aerobic activity may trigger mechanisms similar to centering devices used in meditation. Moreover, the activity of dance itself may substitute for negative stress-related habits or catalyze a different attitude toward one's situation.

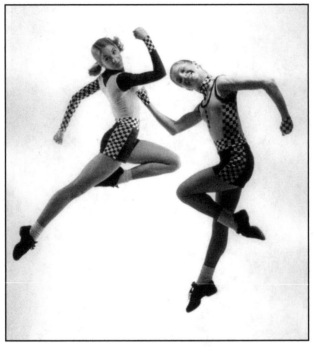

**Figure 2.4. Euphoria (Photo of Adrienne and Ashley Canterna by Chris Dame)**

State anxiety, a transitory condition of foreboding about an impending disaster that may be real, imaginary, or even unknown, responds to habitual aerobic activity. Strenuousness, which varies from person to person, is a major determinant in the response. But twenty minutes of sustained heavy breathing is the minimum amount of time required for an effect to occur.[16] Certain chemistry can dissipate stress. Various endorphins (beta-endorphin and beta-lipotropin) produced by the brain, anterior pituitary gland, and other tissues released into the body as a result of dancing can have a morphine-like effect in reducing the perception of pain.

Dance is a release, a relaxation that dissipates tension build-up. The Dogon of Mali describe their rapid *gona* dance movement as a "relief, like vomiting."[17] Quick motion in dance is especially intoxicating and blissful.[18] Dancing may also be a form of sublimation, a redirection of energy otherwise spent. People dancing in warm, humid climates may experience simple heat exhaustion from diminished cardiac output as a consequence of increased blood flow to the muscles and skin. The result may be a feeling of dizziness or fainting (syncope) accompanied by a fast pulse and often cool skin.[19] Coupled with a person's religious beliefs of spiritual possession, this experience appears to be associated with trance states that may serve to prevent or lead to healing of stress.

Research suggests that tension reduction following exercise lasts longer than passive therapies such as meditation and distraction.[20] Dance can increase the levels of brain chemicals norepinephrine and serotonin, chemicals that decrease in cases of stress-induced depression. Dance can provide remedial neuromuscular action by lengthening, thinning, and relaxing the muscles that tighten in stress reactions.

### Counterindications for Dance

There are situations in which dance as an intervention treatment for stress might be counterindicated for the same reasons that running, another aerobic form of exercise, might be counterindicated.[21] For a patient with severe depression and a fragile ego, a failure in the dance experience might precipitate an intensive depressive episode or a suicidal gesture. Obsessive-compulsives, anorexics, bulimics, and competitive workaholics might turn dancing into a destructive experience. The conclusion to this book notes some prescriptive and proscriptive research findings concerning indications and counterindications for dance.

## Dance: A Stressor Itself

The role of dance in stress patterns for amateurs and professionals depends on whether the dancer perceives the experience as enjoyable or not (the difference may not be noticeable to an outside observer). When a person's behavior is motivated by the pleassure found in dance, self-confidence, contentment, and feelings of solidarity with others accrue. However, if external pressures or rewards motivate the dancer, the individual may experience insecurity, frustration, and a sense of alienation.

### Criticism

Dance may be a stressor for observers. Often a libel-free medium for social criticism or commentary of persons involved in sensitive or contentious issues, dancers may target individuals or groups. The performers may find some relief from a problem by getting it off their chests. Masquerades and possession dances tend to hide the identity of the dancer, who transforms into a supernatural being and can speak out with religious cover, while the target of complaint undergoes stress.

For Western dance, as for other performing arts, the theater is an arena in which to play with sensitive themes without the penalties that accrue to a person's expression of them in everyday life. Themes enacted in dance often bear upon the raw nerves of an individual's personal or group conflicts to create stress for the dancer or onlooker. For further criticism of dance, see chapters 3, 6, and 8.

### Getting to the Dance
Because many dance classes and theaters in the West are located in congested urban areas, the effort to physically get to and from a dance activity may be stressful. An individual may have to organize a busy life in order to fit dance in. Fighting traffic to reach a studio or theater on time, getting something to eat on the way, and finding parking if one drives are part of the effort. If a person has children, arranging for a babysitter can present obstacles to overcome. Obtaining tickets can be difficult if a performance is popular; numerous phone calls must be made when box-office or ticket-sales lines are busy. The high price of theater tickets may stress spectators as well as their economic resources. And then, if the spectator dislikes the performance, stress is compounded.

During my study of the performer-audience connection,[22] an audience member hostile to abstract postmodern dance wrote on an interview form: "A rip-off . . . I think having to pay to see a performance like this is absolutely a SHAM! I am including my name, etc., for I wish to discuss this further and would like a refund." A couple complained to me that they had come for entertainment. They had invested money, including transportation expenses, and time, only to be disappointed.

### Amateur Dancing
As in learning processes generally, some people may be intimidated by an instructor or fearful of making fools of themselves before the teacher or their classmates. This is especially the case for amateur dancers. Sometimes in a social dance setting, an individual may experience rejection from potential partners, or partners may lack coordination or miscommunicate. Stepping on a partner's toes or being stepped on sends the wrong message. For more on the subject of amateur dancing, see chapter 10.

### Professional Dance Career
Artistic development with a minimum amount of stress is an ideal that dance participants desire. Professional dance training may be stressful for the same reasons that amateur dancing has stressful repercussions. In addition, the dance career has its own stressors. Inadequate training is a serious stressor. Besides being highly competitive, dance is fraught with risks of physical and emotional injury, which may end one's performing career. In some technically demanding

dance genres (for example, ballet), dancers must continually work their bodies far beyond normal use and are physically aged by age thirty. Many dancers suffer performance anxiety, what is referred to as stage fright. Because contemporary dancers are expected to be thin, individuals who lack the good fortune to have the body metabolism that enables them to eat whatever they fancy without gaining weight often experience stress associated with dieting, eating disorders, and being rejected for roles because of their weight. Strong personalities sometimes experience stress from their roles as tools of the choreographer and consequently fear losing their individuality. Dancers, especially in ballet, must cope with a brief performing career and then a transition to a new career.

Professional dancers often have economic stressors: not having enough weeks of performance to be eligible for unemployment, low salaries, a lack of savings, problems of obtaining insurance coverage, scheduling a second job[23] and stress related to touring. Teachers and company directors face the difficulty of finding spaces for training, rehearsal, and performance in times of rising rents at the same time that performance itself is limited in its productivity. Other stress factors are the conflicts between economic dilemmas and artistic goals faced by dance companies, administrators, and artistic directors. Racial discrimination had been a problem in dancer recruitment and bookings, but dance companies are more concerned with body size, ability, and height for partnering. Dance scholar Brenda Dixon Gottschild has found that there is not a black dancing body—nor a white dancing, or other dancing body.[24] For more on professional dance careers, see chapter 11.

## Cultural Sensitivity

Dancing in a therapy session or classroom in which the therapist or teacher disregards cultural values creates stress. Western therapy, modern dance, contact improvisation, and dance in kindergarten through twelfth grade emphasize individual self-expression in dance. Anglo-Americans value the freedom to shape their own destiny and consider self-actualization for everyone to be unlimited. In contrast, members of some groups find individuality antithetical to their value systems.[25] The Chinese are "accustomed to containing expressive behavior."[26] Many American Indian groups value anonymity—accepting group sanctions and routinized patterns. Some Latinos tend to esteem routinized life and obedience to the will of God. Moreover, the emphasis on autonomy may appear to promise more than an individual can realize within the contraints of the broader society and economy.

If the cultural group to which the client belongs believes the cause of stress is external to the self, a therapist needs to ascertain what the perceived boundaries of the self are. If illness is punishment for transgression, then it is necessary to understand what is considered deviance and what amends should be made. If disease is believed to result from sin, then expiation is necessary for a cure.

Styles of interaction differ between Anglo and Mescalero Apache Indian patterns, and teachers and therapists might provide familiarity and security for the Mescalero by drawing upon their cultural patterns.[27] These change agents could provide role models for learning by observation rather than calling out rules, as in Anglo culture, use the disciplinary tactic of removing an offender from the group rather than reprimanding the person verbally, permit physical closeness and group work among relatives rather than having individual activities, and organize people in circles rather than rows and rectangular shapes.

In the 1970s, Mexican Americans had distinct notions about styles of behavior in therapy. Curing behavior was expected to involve direct eye contact, prompt diagnosis, religious sanction, appreciation and respect for the patient's self-diagnosis, respect for the patient's beliefs, minimal physical contact, treatment in the family context, and consideration of male dominance over the female.[28] These notions are usually counter to Anglo practice. Thus its success in serving Mexican Americans is hampered.

Catalysts for the use of therapeutic dance vary among groups that are often thought of as having the same lifestyle. As an example, among southwest American Indians, Apachean and Pima peoples have held ceremonies when stressful conditions occur. Most Navajo Indian dances are prayers to cure a particular person's illness.[29] On the other hand, Pueblo groups have ceremonials, the occurrence of which is governed by the calendar, that are intimately involved with the creative cycle, production of rain, and concepts of "like cures like" (as in sympathetic magic). Many American Indians on their reservations use traditional methods of dealing with stress. Even American Indians in urban areas who are fully assimilated into society away from the reservation might better respond to therapies that bear similarity to their respective traditional ways, such as group and sessions arranged by the calendar.

## Stress Management Approaches

Individuals may participate in stress-management programs in a variety of ways: sequentially, at one time or another, or simultaneously in one or more venues. The means of preventing and managing stress are variable and at times even contradictory. In fact, stress may produce a nonpathological cross-resistance. Treating one stressor may increase the body's resistance to others.

Having a healthy lifestyle (such as one that incorporates the exercise of dance and a well-balanced diet) certainly is a way to manage stress. Some religious groups have dances set according to regular calendar events, in addition to other rituals that come into play with specified crises. Such events help followers avoid stress or react to it in a constructive manner. There are approaches that involve action, while others require passivity. The sacred and secular often intersect in healing techniques. Various types of stress-management approaches are not always explicitly named as such. For example, participants in religious rituals that help people cope with stress may regard these actions only as practices prescribed by belief systems related to supernatural entities. Followers of a secular lifestyle that serves to resist or reduce stress, and sometimes to escape it, may be unaware of such benefits.

Another kind of stress-management program is secular therapy that has its roots in ritual dance practices. The shaman, or medicine person, in non-Western dances is an avatar of the dance therapist. Within the secular therapeutic stress-management approach, there are two prominent models, human potential and medical. The latter has two different orientations.

In the human-potential model, the therapist helps the healthy individual to develop her or his own qualities. This self-actualization refers to self-expression, self-fulfillment, and autonomy from external forces. The existential, humanistic psychologies are not concerned with disability but with humankind more broadly.

The human-potential model is similar to the wellness, or holistic health, model. Herein all aspects of the human being—mind, body, and soul—are viewed as interrelated and essential to the others. When these are in balance in relation to an individual's environment, a state of wellness exists. The approach has roots in ancient healing methods. Hippocrates and Galen, ancient Greek physicians, recognized the value of exercise. By the time of the Renaissance, nutrition and exercise were thought to be ways humans could wrest control of their destiny from God's will. In a wellness model, some decision making and responsibility rests with the client.

In contrast with the human-potential, or wellness, model, the typical medical model assumes the client is ill, and the therapist attempts to diagnose and heal individuals by helping them to cope with their specific pathologies. The medical model is most relevant to victims of post-traumatic stress disorder.

## Styles of Intervention

There are various styles of intervention in stress situations. Autogenic, or self-conducted, styles mean that the individual takes the initiative in some way, whether it is to meet his or her god through dance, take a dance class, dance spontaneously, or visit a dance therapist. The individual maintains decision-making authority and responsibility for action. In directive styles, a member of a society, such as a family member, priest, or therapist, who observes stress-ridden behavior will direct or induce the individual to act in a structured way to meet specific goals. Another approach to intervention is evocative therapy, which helps people modify their behavior by indirectly creating favorable conditions for modification but eliciting their self-reflection and leaving change up to them.

More than one style of intervention may be operative at the same time. Each directive style involves interpretation based on the therapist's theoretical system of psychology, whether it is expressed in terms of cosmology, ancestor honor, or Freud's theory of the ego and id.

## Dance Genres

Not only are there variations in relationships between dance and stress, stress-management approaches, and styles of intervention in stress situations, but there are also different dance genres associated with stress-related behavior. In the literature, one finds such oppositions as "primitive" versus theater, classical versus folk, social versus ethnic, and ballet versus modern. However, the categories often are poorly defined and blur together.

Ritual dance is an extraordinary event involving stylized repetitive behavior. It may include practices of magic (sacramental utterances, exorcisms, curses, and blessings that are believed to set in motion some supernatural entity or transcendent power), prayer, or sacrifice. A common goal is to link society and its environment, specifically, extracting goods and services from the supernatural environment for society. Dance is sometimes part of religious expression to worship or honor the deities, conduct supernatural beneficence, effect change, and embody the supernatural through inner transformation and personal possession or through an external transformation as in a masquerade.[30] Steeped in religion, these dance practices bring to life the imaginary work of the invisible supernatural.

There are distinctions in ritual dances based on the kind of participation that is involved. Some dances are dancer initiated. In contrast with the dancer intentionally doing, the dancer may be becoming, that is, being acted upon by the supernatural. Ritual dance, like totemic ideas and myths, appears to be part of a cultural code enabling the human being to order experience, account for its chaos, and explain affective and cognitive realities. Coupling the hedonic and cognitive, dance has the power to create a second world, one of virtual time and space.

Dance is ethnic when it is explicitly linked to the cultural tradition of a group with a sense of identity based upon origins, and its members constitute part of a larger society. Ethnic dance is folk when it is a communal expression; folk dance need not be ethnic, but both may be forms of social, ritual, or theatrical dance. The context of a dance clarifies its type and whether it is a first- or second-existence folk dance. First existence refers to dance as an essential part of life, whereas a second existence refers to a revival or arrangement, perhaps a stage performance.[31] The Russian Mosieyev Dance Company presents folk dances, but it certainly is considered theater dance, second existence folk dance. An ethnic group in the United States may alternatively perform its dance in a member's home at a holiday as a social dance or in a theater for a heterogeneous audience, a first and second existance folk dance, respectively. The lack of clear-cut dance categorizations also appears in regard to classical ballet as an ethnic dance with European origins.[32] However, ballet is no longer European but has become international.

A key purpose of social dance is to provide the opportunity for people to get together and interact. This genre includes popular dance (common in the dominant culture in a heterogeneous setting), ethnic-folk-national dance, and some forms of dance therapy.

Exercise dance refers to dance aerobics, jazzercize, and other forms of bodily exertion that incorporate simple contemporary social dancelike movement patterns with musical accompaniment to make physical fitness activities enjoyable.

Theater dance includes forms of dance that require specialized training and are presented onstage for an audience: thus ballet, modern (the rebellion against classical ballet heralded by Loie Fuller, Isadora Duncan, Ruth St. Denis, and Martha Graham) postmodern dance (the reaction to modern dance led by Merce Cunningham), jazz, tap, and Broadway musicals. Theater dance has limited audience participation; the spectator is distanced from the dancer.

Therapeutic dance activities depend upon the client's movement skill and vocabulary. Sometimes dance therapy uses only body movement and would not be recognized as dance per se by the average person in the United States.

Having presented some dance genres that are involved in stress management, and having noted that the categories are not clear cut, we should be aware of the processes of change that have contributed to the phenomenon of dance. Dance genres are always transforming and may also fulfill different functions at different times. People borrow from each other. Sometimes one group's dances are imposed on another.

# Filling in the Sketch

I have sketched connections between dance and stress and will now fill in the sketch with illustrative cases of dance as a stress vaccine or stress buster drawn from ethnographic, historical, clinical, and experimental research. Because the available data related to the dance-stress connection vary, so too does the discussion of illustrative cases vary in depth.

Chapters 1 and 2 presented a theoretical framework for dance and stress. Although the typology of relationships is based on a survey of case material, the cases that follow do not always fit neatly into one or another of the categories. Consequently, the following chapters are organized in terms of illustrative examples of ritual, social, ethnic, amateur, and professional dance genres and stress that are clustered by specific mode of action or problems addressed: meeting the supernatural (chapter 3) or acting in other religiously motivated ways (chapters 4 and 5), resolving conflicts in the secular arena (chapter 6), and confronting political and economic changes catalyzed by the clash of old or new dance group patterns (chapter 7).

Some common themes occur in both parts II and III. Death, for example, is a universally stressful event that people attempt to cope with in religious dance practices as well as in secular dance. Feared not just by individuals but by societies, the cessation of life wrenches and dislocates part of the fabric of social relationships. The more important the person, the greater the number and range of ties that are snapped. People must reorganize themselves after the demise of someone at the center of a cluster of social relations. The death of others holds intimations of our own mortality and creates other kinds of anxiety and fear.

Contemporary psychologists recognize the need for bereaved individuals to have some help for a year or more in dealing with grief and coming to terms with the loss of someone close. We see ourselves reflected in the daily response of our partners. The mourning process involves both the mind and the body. Stress is commonly marked by denial, anger, degrees of depression, and eventual acceptance.

People can get stuck in bereavement-linked depressions. The stress of bereavement tends to be disruptive to one of the body's basic systems of stress regulation, namely, the hypothalamic-pituitary-adrenal axis, which is activated in response to a threat of danger.[33] Therefore, preventative and redressive action is needed and taken through various dance genres to cope with the death of people—and also communities.

# PART II

# HISTORICAL AND NON-WESTERN DANCE-STRESS RELATIONS

Throughout time, people have danced to cope with stress in non-Western cultures and Western minority cultures, both past and present. The examples in the next five chapters offer a cross-cultural perspective that may lead to innovation in your own life and culture, effectiveness in dealing with others, and further understanding of meaning in dance movement. Recall that the relatively new term *stress* has become the umbrella for concepts like conflict, frustration, trauma, anomie, alienation, anxiety, and depression.

Our panorama considers how people, mainly communally, meet their gods and demons with praise and appeal, possession, masking, and exorcism to prevent stress and to achieve healing. The spotlight turns to ways people have engaged tarantula bites for the bite itself and also as an excuse to respond to other stressors. Dance mediated the devastating Black Death that occurred over a period of many centuries. Pestilence called for village purification driven by dance. The stress of a repressed sex drive found its outlet in the dance, which was also used as a means of reducing the stress of life transitions, from birth to death, and managing conflict. Political conquest creates stressors of lost land, group dignity, and self-identity. Social and political stressors lead groups to congregate and deal with their woes through dance. In this part of the book, we look at how dance has been a vehicle to help to deal with such problems.

# CHAPTER THREE

~

# Meeting the Gods and Demons

## Praise and Appeal

Religious belief systems often offer explanations for stressful events and be-havior. People may believe that gods cause famine and spirits make people ill or difficult to get along with. Dance is frequently part of general ritual scenes, social milieus, and specific practices that are presumed to appease the divinities or exorcise demons or malevolence caused by spirits. Honoring supernatural entities to preclude their angry creation of stressors for natural beings, dance is a prophylactic strategy. Thus humans perform dance to re-vere, as a gesture of fellowship or hospitality, and to show respect. A remedial approach is to dance to propitiate or beseech supernatural entities to change stressful conditions, or to dance to expurgate the stressor. Dance may also be a religiously sanctioned "time out" (even euphoric state) to gain relief from a stressful situation. In healing rituals, the shaman, priest, or equiv-alent applies part of the mythic world to the patient's particular circum-stance.

There are numerous illustrations of religious dance practices that serve to resist or to reduce stress. The following approaches are stylistically autogenic. The Old Testament refers to rejoicing before God with a person's entire being. Thus the Jews dance to praise their God in sublime adoration and to express thanks for his beneficence. The Kalabari of Nigeria say that men make the gods great. Fervent dancing adds to a deity's ability to aid the worshippers—and just as surely, cutting off the dancing will render the deity impotent or at the least break off contact with erstwhile worshippers.[1]

The Sandawe of Tanzania believe the moon to be a supreme being who is either beneficent or destructive. Identifying with the moon, the dancers adopt stylized signs of moon stances to metaphorically conduct supernatural beneficence. The moonlit erotic dance in which couples embrace tightly and mimic the act of fertilization is assumed to promote fertility.[2] Numerous groups in Africa are dominated by males. Yet the men often honor the female gods and their living and ancestral representatives. For example, among the Yoruba of Nigeria, men masquerade as women to attract the females' goodwill. Women are believed to have secrets, life-giving power, and also witchlike powers, including the ability to cause male impotency. The dance is meant to eliminate the negative aspects of female power and replace them with fecundity, maternity, and general well-being.[3]

Dance may be a medium to reverse a debilitating condition caused by the supernatural. When the Gogo men of Tanzania fail in their ritual responsibility to control human and animal fertility, disorder reigns. The women then become the only active agents in rituals addressed to righting the wrong. Dressed as men, they dance violently with spears to drive away contamination.[4]

Other religiously motivated actions to cope with stress are possession, masking, and exorcism. These modes may occur independently or in combination, and they involve several psychological processes, especially catharsis.

## Possession

Through the dance, a person may invite possession by temporarily giving the self to a supernatural being and thereby achieve a consciousness of identity or ritual connection. Experiencing an inner transformation that allows the dancer to embody the supernatural, she or he performs identifiable and specific patterns and conventional signs communicating to the entire group present that the supernatural is enacting its particular role in managing stress in human life. Thus fear of the supernatural entity's indifference is allayed.

Cult members, diviners, medicine men, mediums, and shamans are among those who invite the gods to possess their bodies. The possessed then act on another person's behalf. In spiritualist sects such as the Umbanda, Candomblé, Tango, Quimbanda, and Catimbo in Brazil, participants use possession to temporarily escape from daily worries and gain liberation from blocked emotional tensions.[5]

Among the Irigwe of Nigeria, the traditional marriage custom calls for both men and women to marry several spouses from different tribal areas and for the women to shift residence among husbands several times during her lifetime. Perhaps to relieve the stress "arising from their repeated separations from loved ones and to achieve social integration to compensate . . . for the repeated separations." Irigwe women often become possessed during spirit cult dances. They "cry, speak in tongues, and flail about after the frenetic drumming, dancing, singing; and rattling leg irons had induced a dissociated state in them . . . giving vent without castigation to their repressed feelings."[6]

In Korea, the most elaborate shaman ritual, the *kut*, aims to bring good fortune, to heal, or to send off the dead. Following a sequence in which certain deities appear, the dance is a means to invoke the gods and encourage their descent into the shaman. The female shaman (who outnumbers male practitioners in male-dominated Korea) is a specialist for housewives who experience gender-related stress.[7] In essence, the shaman gives a "women's party" held by and for women. Claiming to see the deities and beckon them to speak through her lips, she puts on a particular god's costume. To drum accompaniment, the shaman sings an invocation and then with outstretched arms dances gracefully until a burst of drumbeats and a series of leaps reveal the descent of the gods. Kicks and flailing arms announce that the gods are strong. After a few shamans have invoked several of the sponsoring family's household gods, the shamans rest. During this interval, one after another of the women of the household and their relatives and neighbors puts on the shaman's costume and dances to receive her personal god.

In the invasion-possession dance, often a metaphor and signal of social pathology or personal maladjustment, the supernatural being overwhelms an individual who is causing some form of malaise, illness, or personal or group misfortune. The dance exorcises the being, thus freeing the possessed individual from stress and ameliorating the irksome situation. Meeting the wishes of a spirit as part of directive exorcism usually imposes obligations on the possessed's relatives.

A Moroccan Sufi brotherhood, the Hamadsha, perform the *hadra* ecstatic dance in order to cure an individual who has been struck by the devil or possessed by one. The ritual helps to relieve anxiety, physical tension, and emotional stress.[8] When bothered by paresthetic pains (feelings of numbness, prickling, and tingling), cult members find relief and a sense of revitalization in the dancing and trance.

Attack by a *jinn* (spirit) causes facial or other paralysis, convulsions, or sudden (hysterical) blindness or deafness. Medical anthropologists Ann McElroy and Patricia Townsend note that

> excessive anxiety and hyperventilation can cause these symptoms. . . . People
> attacked by a *jinn* often recover from these symptoms overnight if they dance;
> however, they may experience aftereffects of . . . a lack of energy. Using our

knowledge of the [stress syndrome] stages of alarm, resistance, and exhaustion, we can see that respiratory alkalosis and paralysis are an alarm reaction to the stressor of anxiety, a recurrent psychological feature of the Moroccans who belong to the Hamadsha. Through a variety of sensory overload techniques, the dancers induce stress, which brings on a stage of resistance to the initial psychosomatic illness of paralysis. The depression and temporary fatigue experienced after trance are analogous to the strain evidenced in the stage of exhaustion; since the initial stressor is removed, however, there is little serious danger that this strain will lead to permanent damage.[9]

The dancers seek a good relationship with a jinn, usually the she-demon 'A'isha Quandisha. During the ritual she may emerge from the ground and dance alongside the human performers. She causes the dancers' heads to swell, their hair to stand on end, and their scalps to itch. Slashing her own head is an example to them. As the dance progresses, the participants become entranced and, in imitation of the saint Sidi Ali's servant, slash at their heads. The flow of blood is believed to calm the spirit. Certain of the Hamadsha form teams that perform the *hadra* professionally for the stricken and the sick.

The Malays believe God has a cure for all ills, and sometimes the remedy includes dance, especially when spirits have caused an illness.[10] A healthy person is protected from harm by the universal spirit that dwells in all creations and the Inner Winds governing the individual talent and personality inherited from his or her parents. However, if strong Winds are not expressed, they accumulate in the body and cause physical and emotional pain, and even an imbalance of humors, leaving the person vulnerable to the depredations of spirits. This requires external spirits to be exorcised through a séance during which shaman and patient dance. The shaman changes personas, all of which are identified by their movments and postures, as well as by their voices and speech. He dances slowly and stately, bending and swaying his body like a branch waving in the breeze. His gestures have specific meanings; a palm facing toward the sky bids the spirits to remain calm; his arm outstretched and bent at the elbow, palm outward and with lightly raised fingers, requests protection; a closed fist with thumb outside brought up to the mouth or temple signifies his recall of magical knowledge.[11] When a shaman dances before his patient in the persona of a spirit who has agreed to be helpful, the shaman may grab the patients's head or shoulders to pull the oppressive vapor from the patient's body into his own hands and then release it into the air. The patient's trance prior to dancing allows her or him to open the inner self. Individuals may experience invited or invasion possession by a supernatural potency.

Part of ritual healing, trance dancing among the Temiar in Malaysia commands attention with its narrative, sensory embodiment. Issues of health as well as colonialism and modernity (deforestation, Islamic religious evange-lism, economic transformation) create schisms in personal and community life. Ritual healing deals with the distress of individuals and mitigates the effects of contact with foreigners as it helps to reestablish cultural integrity and resolve new types of illness/soul loss associated with disruption and dis-location. The souls of human and nonhuman entities are dialectically differ-entiated into benevolent and malevolent opposing forces, which the Temiar attempt to control through dream and trance. The dream process involves the head-soul spirit of the dreamer meeting with a portion of souls of entities (such as trees, river rapids, and deceased humans), who upon declaring to become their spirit guide bestow songs upon them. In the ceremonial per-formance setting that follows, the spiritual link effectually transforms the dreamer into a medium of the spirit guide, acquiring its voice, vision, and knowledge.[12]

Among the !Kung Bushmen of Namibia, prolonged dancing to women's singing heats up and activates *n/um*, a therapeutic substance that resides in the stomachs of medicine men, who are renowned dancers. These healers derive their power for remediation and protection from sickness and death from this overwhelming potency within their bodies, which exudes in the form of sweat. The ceremonial curing dance, and the medicine that can be transferred from these dancers to patients, is called for during crisis situations, and it occurs spontaneously for good measure.

This Bushmen healing dance is both a case of people escaping stress and seeking stress for religious therapeutic purposes. People come together as a unit to sing, clap, and dance. "They are doing something together that gives them pleasure, they become enlivened in spirit and body, and for a time they gain freedom from the arduous unremitting search for food and escape their usual anxieties that fill their days."[13] The dancing may last from twelve to thirty-six hours, with individuals participating in four- to six-hour shifts.

The stimulation of physical movement, the constant rhythm of the music, sensory overload, hyperventilation in breathing, and autosuggestion facilitate trance. When *n/um* boils through the sensory overload of the curing ritual and its stress of excessive stimulation, the men enter an altered state of con-sciousness, which the Bushmen call half-death, and we call trance. The !Kung experience dizziness, disorientation, hallucinations, and muscle spasms, symp-toms we would normally view as alarming evidence of illness.[14] The medicine man "in trance absorbs the patient's disease into his own body and lets it run its full course inside his body."[15]

Contact with white immigrants from South Africa and black ranchers who settled in the Ghazi district was disruptive to the San Bushmen. They experienced the stressors of unemployment, poverty, hunger, and new diseases as well as a degrading self-image. The prominence of suffering has led to the trance dancer's unprecedented social importance. In contrast with the hunting-gathering Bushman, the farming Bushman trance dancer assumes professional status and achieves wealth and prestige. Moreover, armed with heroic and mystic power, the dancer revitalizes the Bushman culture and self-image.[16]

In a number of Christian denominations, dancers may become possessed during church services through, as they say, "feeling the spirit." For example, members of the black American Pentecostal Church of Holy Christ in Pittsburgh, Pennsylvania, believe God is the Father of Christ, who was conceived by the Holy Ghost and born of the Virgin Mary. Dying for the sins of humans, Christ went to heaven to prepare a place for them and left the Holy Ghost for their comfort. On the day of Pentecost, the Holy Ghost descended to the apostles and gave them the "quickening powers" of speaking in tongues, dancing, and other manifestations of spiritual possession. Dance is thus treated as a divine occurrence, a revelation of God to those upon whom he has bestowed the Holy Ghost.[17]

At Mt. Pisgah Missionary Baptist Church in Dallas, on the twenty-fifth anniversary of the Senior Men's Choir, I observed the fervor of the church service reach a high emotional pitch. Individuals in the pews shouted, "Amen," "Preach it, honey," "Yes, sir," "Get on with it." They cried, nodded heads back and forth, swayed sideward, raised their palms upward, shaked, clapped their hands, and danced to the accompaniment in a gospel rhythm (similar to the blues and boogie) of the choir, pianist, and organist. While dancing, some women collapsed into the arms of male ushers. God showed his presence to help the faithful deal with stress.

## Masking

Sacred masquerade dances have stress-related features common to possession dances. Both forms of ritual dance allow people to separate themselves from a problem by distancing or through diversion from stress. The elicited religious and spiritual direction provides sanction and legitimacy for secular actions and allows performers and audience members to transact social relationships with less stress than in everyday life.

Masquerade dances are part of a people's intercourse with the supernatural world. The dancer embodies a supernatural entity through invited external transformation. Beneath the mask, a dancer is believed to undergo change, becoming the supernatural. Under religious auspices, the dancer is freed from everyday restrictions and consequently can present critical messages that might otherwise produce stressful social friction or hostility.

For example, the Nigerian Nsukka Igbo council of elders employ masked dancers representing an *omabe* spirit cult whenever there is difficulty in enforcing law and order.[18] A Chewa man residing with his wife and mother-in-law might resort to the male masked *nyau* dance to mediate between himself and a mother-in-law, whom he dislikes for making constant demands on him. When he dons his mask of the *chirombo* (beast), he enjoys the immunity it bestows upon him. He directs obscene language against the mother-in-law, and she may take no action against him. The mother-in-law usually reduces her demands after the dance.[19] Beyond the dancer's release of energy generated in the fight-or-flight stress response, catharsis, and working through, the dance event effects change in the person causing the stress.

Socially sanctioned ritual abuse with ribald and lewd movements and gesture in a highly charged atmosphere occurs in the Ivory Coast Bedu masked dance. The Nafana people believe that through these acts participants are purged of whatever negative emotions they may harbor.[20] Thus they resist and reduce stress.

## Exorcism and Healing

Possession and masquerade dances may occur in tandem; that is, masked dancers may become possessed. In Sinhalese Buddhist healing rites the exorcist, in a directive and evocative style, attempts to sever the relationship between a patient and malign demons and ghosts in order to reduce or eliminate stress. Emotional tension builds up progressively in the exorcist's performance of various masked dance sequences. These generate power that reaches out and embraces and then enters the healer and/or the patient. Their bodies become the demonic spirit's vehicle, constitute evidence of its control, and convince spectators of the need for a change in social relations, which will transform the patient from ill to healthy. Exorcism works to build the ideal social hierarchical order. The dance is a public validation first that the patient has fallen under a demon's control and second that a cure has been achieved.

The healing rite of the Great Cemetery Demon, Mahasona, is performed in the vicinity of the town of Galle in the southern area of Sri Lanka.[21] The chief participants are the members of the urban working class and rural peasantry. Associated specifically with the subordinate and weak, the healing rite has a disproportionate number of female victims. The Sinhalese view women as subordinate to men, yet also "central in the cultural order and the most sensitive to disturbances in it."[22] Exorcists appear in the guise of women in

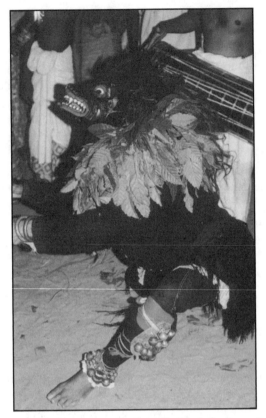

**Figure 3.1.   Sinhalese Demon Healing Rite (Photo by Bruce Kapferer)**

the main dance episodes to attract the demons and thereby to ensnare them in their own demonic natural passion and make them prisoners of their own lust. "Exorcist female attire is symbolic of the mediation of nature and culture in the identity of the female and the vulnerability of women to the attack and control by the demonic. It is during the dance, held at a time when demonic power is in its ascendancy, that an exorcist-dancer will become possessed by the demon."[23] Transvestism is not the point. Rather, "the strength and authority of the male lies behind and within the female. During the dance, the demonic enters into the male body of a dancer dressed as a female. Trapped in a male body, which is also healthy and nonafflicted, the demonic can be controlled and expelled."[24]

Exorcists are from a special caste, *berava*. Aspiring exorcists seek out recognized exponents, with whom they study. Apprenticeships beginning as early as six or seven years of age usually begin with dance instruction and then proceed to the art of drumming, intoning mantras (spells), and singing. Exorcists assist each other with performances.

The exorcist discovers the malevolent supernatural agents involved in an illness and also uncovers the social events surrounding the patient and others who have exposed the patient to demonic attack or evince demonic malevolence. "A disturbance of the body is also a disturbance of the mind, and *vice versa*."[25] Stress is obviously a critical cause. Extreme emotional states, especially fear, including anger, envy, jealousy, grief, and acute sexual desire are symptomatic of demonic illness.[26] Exorcists typically trace its onset to the patient's experience of sudden fright or fear, whether in dreams or mysterious figures in the night. The patient's experience may be an autogenic call for help.

The decision to have an exorcism is not undertaken lightly. Moreover, demonic agency in illness can be dangerous to those in contact with the patient. "Knowledge that an individual is a demonic victim can lead other members of a neighborhood to reduce their interaction with a patient and a patient's household."[27] For the treatment, patients and their immediate family require the material support and cooperation of other kin and neighbors. In the case of Asoka's illness, the agreement to hold the exorcism was more than a consequence of the severity of her physical symptoms. The decision reflected for her kin a set of social difficulties related to conflict over land and property that they were encountering.[28] Demonic attacks gain prominence in the context of disruption and fragmentation in the social order. A spectacular combination of sound, song, smell, dance, and drama, the "show" of demonic behavior performed throughout the night makes manifest to the senses of patients and onlookers the real intention of demons, which then become accessible to remedial action and stress reduction. To disclose is to expose to therapeutic action, since the unknown is dangerous. Demons seek to hide themselves from reality, from exposure of their true place in the cosmic hierarchy. When Mahasona is revealed in his masked representations, demons can be humiliated, mocked into their proper place in the scheme of things, and cease to be awesome. "Caught out," they have nowhere to go except into ridiculous disgrace.

When the demons are made inferior to humans and the divine through danced comic action, the fear and terror of the demons can be laughed away. In parallel fashion, the structure and contexts of everyday life are also made light of. Exorcists and onlookers enjoin the patient to participate in the comic action. The humor, a tool in coping with stress, is crucial to treating a patient, who is brought out of demonic obsession/possession and restored to the world of social relationships.

Exorcism restores the individual to a sense of well-being.[29] The process involves a distancing that allows individuals to stand outside their own subjectivity, constitute themselves as objects, and then reconstitute themselves in a state of well-being.

The dancing episodes and the patient's entrancement constitute evidence in the views of the exorcist and audience that the patient has fallen under the demon's control. With elaborate dance, the exorcists win the confidence of observers in their skills to overcome the demon. The comic mocking signifies that the demons are denied a position of dominance, whereupon the patient has the opportunity to be identified as no longer subject to demonic attack.

Dance draws performers and spectators into the demonic and divine realm of its creation. The exorcists understand their dances to constitute the greatest elaboration of supernatural force.[30] Exorcists and onlookers believe the dancers become one with the forces they generate.

> Like the gods, the demons are presented with ceremony . . . the magnificent dance is in their honour. But as they are called and celebrated, so are the gods, whose authority and purity will destroy, control, and repel the demons. In the dance the dancer resides the divine. . . . The entire rite . . . can be seen as the elaborate springing of a demonic trap, a means for refixing the demons in a cosmic order which they have momentarily escaped.[31]

## Afterword

In meeting gods and demons made manifest in the dance medium, individuals often resist, reduce, or escape stress. In dancing to appease the supernatural, to appeal to reverse a debilitating condition, or to exorcise malevolence, performers may develop physical fitness to ward off the debilitating effects of fatigue, old age, and pressures of daily life. The ritual of healing, validated through the associated dance, mediates through religious legitimacy the social relations that caused an individual or group distress or illness. There seems to be an implicit awareness that a person's or community's stress is affected by interactions with the environment. Much of the dancing is cathartic and prescriptive working through. Dancing in possession and trance permit a temporary euphoric state and escape from anxiety and depression. Religious beliefs sanction many behaviors contemporary research scientists have found to be effective stress-management techniques.

~

## CHAPTER FOUR

# Shaking Off Poison, Plague, Death, and Sin

History attests to dancing as a response to the stressors of poisonous spider bites, pestilence, plagues, peril, and sexuality—indeed, a wide variety of medical and psychological syndromes. In this chapter, I present four illustrative cases (tarantism, the Black Death, *ketjak,* and Shaker dance). The cases are part of both religious and secular behavior. Although the dance-stress pattern may have a specific initial catalyst, the performance may encompass other stressors as well.

## Tarantism

Tarantism, in which dancing plays a key role in expurgating the venom and curing the bite (real or imaginary) of the tarantula spider, is a hysterical phenomenon related to dancing mania.[1] Medical doctor Justice Friedrich Carl Hecker reported that disorientation from the spider bite left victims susceptible to empassioned dancing to the point of exhaustion at the first tones of familiar melodies.[2] A demand for attention and social support, besides an outlet for pent-up emotions and release of energy mobilized in response to stress characterize the outbreaks of tarantism.

From ethnomusicologist Gilbert Rouget's summary of the literature on tarantism comes the following information.[3] A text dating from 1621 reports that victims of the tarantula bite, "almost moribund because of the venom, moaning, anguished, agonizing, almost bereft of . . . [their] senses, external and internal," could return to their senses upon hearing the sound of musical instruments. Such individuals opened their eyes, pricked up their ears, rose, began to make slight movements with their fingers and toes and then, keeping the rhythm of the melody, began dancing with great liveliness, shaking the body and limbs.[4] This dance agitation released opiumlike pain-killing chemicals or provided distraction that ameliorated stress.

Dancers collapse before as well as after going into trance. During the entire time that the "tarantulee" is entranced, the dance is intended to lead to a collapse until the end, when the person is granted "grace." The perpetual motion is critical in the resolution. The music, with its rhythmical order, unleashes "that most elementary sign of life which is movement, while at the same time, the discipline of the rhythm prevents the movement from sliding into pure psychomotoric convulsions."[5]

Each species of tarantula has its own special tune, although the same dance is always performed. A musical motto was a means of identifying the spider responsible for the possession. In the late nineteenth century, twelve different tarantella themes were used to diagnose tarantulees in Naples, Italy. An ill patient did not know if she had been bitten by a tarantula or by a scorpion. So the musicians who had been summoned began trying out their themes. "At the fourth, the tarantulee immediately began to sigh, and at last, no longer able to resist the call of the dance, she leapt half naked from her bed, without a thought for conventions, and for three days kept up a springthly dance after which she was cured."[6]

A varient of tarantism appears in Sardinia, Italy. Here the mythical creature, the *argia*, causes the patient's poisoning. This creature "is categorized under three distinct species, the nubile, the wife, and the widow, and the treatment of the poisoned person differs according to the type of *argia* that bit him or her."[7]

Tarantism, long regarded as a spectacular form of therapy, has been variously interpreted. Some scholars see it "as simply one element in a vast system of symbolic representations one might call astrological in nature." Others see it "as a form of exorcism functioning within the psychoanalytic logic of a religion based on remorse." Both perspectives "also associate tarantism as a religious phenomenon with possession cults as a whole, but they do so with what one might term repugnance."[8]

Marius Schneider[9] sees a system of mystical correspondence between nature and human, among the elements, astrological signs, the seasons, and sounds as the cause of the spider dance. This correspondence functions "as a form of therapy acting both on the level of accidental reality (that of the illness produced by the spider's bite) and on the level of permanent reality (that of the struggle between life and death, summer and winter, stillness and movement, renewal and decay). Within the overall configuration of these mystic correspondences, musical sounds, musical instruments, and dance steps occupy a well-defined position. It is by virtue of this position, and of the power it con-fers upon them, that music and dance ensure the triumph of recovery, which should simply be seen as an example of the victory of life." Rouget's critique is that the symbolic system Schneider describes has never actually been observed and nothing proves that the elements that make it up have ever constituted a whole.[10]

Thirteen years after Schneider's work appeared, De Martino came to a totally different interpretation based on team fieldwork conducted in Salento in 1959. He considers tarantism as a "minor religious form" of exorcism, the origins of which are likely to be found in the "orgiastic and initiatory cults of classical antiquity." He thinks the actual spider poisoning that the Christian armies experienced during the Crusades catalyzed the birth of the tarantula symbol. The activities surrounding it became an institution that functioned on a "mythico-ritual horizon of recapture and reintegration in relation to critical moments of human existence, with a marked preference for the crisis of puberty, the theme of the forbidden eros, and the conflicts of adolescence, within the framework of a peasant lifestyle."[11]

One of the dance figures is an imitation of the spider's movements. With the tarantulee's back to the ground, body arched, movement takes place on all fours. According to a seventeenth-century account, some tarantulees let themselves hang outdoors from trees by ropes or indoors from a rope affixed to a ceiling. More than mere imitation, De Martino interprets this figure as symbolic of the swing of hanged virgins and Phaedra's hanging, and thus a sign of frustrated, unhappy, or thwarted female passions. It is also symbolic, he says, of being rocked in a mother's arms and then being temporarily abandoned.

Rouget, however, argues that this best-known example of trance in all of Europe "turns out to be nothing more than a particular form of possession." The essential thing is not exactly what the dancers are trying to rid themselves of, but rather how they do it. The dance is placed under the sign of Saint Paul, whose chapel serves as a "theater" for the tarantulees' public meetings. The spider seems to be constantly interchangeable with Saint Paul; the female tarantulees dress as "brides of Saint Paul" and even today sing, "Say where the tarantula stung you / Underneath the hem of my skirt/ . . . Oh my Saint Paul of the tarantulas / Who stings all the girls / And makes them saints."[12]

Tarantism, as in other forms of possession, involved entrancement during which the dancer indulges in extravagant behavior, including movement like a spider. Healing from the tarantula bite is the intended result of tarantism. This, however, provided a providential alibi, for the Church of Rome could never tolerate the existence of an overt possession cult, a form of ritualized therapy. Women who give themselves up to possession practices in tarantism, however, were not sinners but unfortunate victims of the spider, and the music and dance mechanically expelled the venom. The tarantism also provided a woman with a way to behave like an hysteric in public, in accordance with a model recognized by all, thereby freeing her from inner misfortune and relief from hard work, childbearing, and an overbearing husband. Rouget sees this "coming out of herself" and communicating with society "as a response to a need for communication."[13]

There is ambiguity in tarantism, for although the bite is most frequently imaginary, it can sometimes be real. In the latter instance, the toxicity causes pain, difficulty in standing, muscular rigidity, trembling, sometimes sexual arousal, and a sensation of burning and tingling in the soles of the feet. Besieged by depression, anxiety, and a sense of impending death, the patient then becomes agitated and hallucinatory, and, consequently, susceptible to dancing to exhaustion upon hearing the first notes of favorite melodies played by wandering musicians. The desire to free oneself from suffering was an invitation to dance. In tarantism, the symbolic and the real coincide. Although the purpose is sometimes to chase out the venom, it is also to expel what it symbolizes.

Irrespective of the different interpretations, we can conclude that the ecstatic attack of tarantism furnished a means of ameliorating or escaping stress. Tarantism may be commemorated in annual recurrences. When a person is poisoned, the dancing may induce stress that detracts from the stress of the venom. Tarantism had a broader reach than a spider bite, the initial catalyst. Sometimes tarantism was a way to deal with stresses of life transitions and conflicts about sexuality. The action of tarantism certainly calls attention to the individual, who intentionally or otherwise may try to resist, reduce, or escape the stress. In the ritual, the musicians provide psychological support, as do observers, who receive messages of adversity as well as empathize with the physical behavior of catharsis, release, or escape through vigorous movement.

A literary example of the tarantism phenomenon comes from Ibsen's *A Doll's House*. Anthropologist Thomas F. Johnston reminded me that the husband forces his unwilling wife to dance the tarantula before assembled guests. She eventually asserts her independence.

## Black Death and Poison

Medieval Europe was an economically harsh and morally complex world with a largely preliterate society. In a society dominated by the Christian church, the world was believed to be fought over by God and the devil. Terror of death and anxieties about the incessant feuds of barons and the repressiveness of state feudalism provoked the compulsion to dance. Dances were a means to cope with daily stress, especially the high mortality rate and short life span. Then came the ravages of the pandemic of a disease transmitted from black rat fleas to humans—but thought to be God's punishment for moral depravity and grave sins. Sins included allowing people who did not worship Christ or God in a way the community did to remain in the community.[14] Because many people did not believe God would punish them so severely, they claimed Jews and other "enemies of Christendom" poisoned their wells. They persecuted these people.

The Black Death (1347–1353) spread by trade and travel by land and sea from China to Greenland, Siberia to India, North Africa and the Middle East, to the southern Balkans, Russia, Hungary, Italy, Spain, France, Belgium, Switzerland, Britain, Norway, Denmark, Sweden, Austria, Germany, and the Netherlands.[15] The plague pressed its relentless advance with great swiftness, often advancing several miles in a single day.[16] The disease got its name from the deep purple, almost black, spots it left on a victim's skin just prior to death. Flea bites left buboes, boils resulting from swollen lymph nodes, usually in the groin and armpits, and abscesses, pustules, and carbuncles. The plague infection in the bloodstream caused chills, fevers, prostration, damage to organs, hemorrhaging of blood vessels, gangrene, and bleeding from the nose and ears. Pneumonic plague, transmitted interpersonally by blood droplets expelled when victims coughed or sneezed, caused hemorrhaging and feverish red spots. Thirty to sixty percent of the population, twenty-five million people, were killed by the bubonic plague. It erupted periodically over the next three centuries.

Dancing created an eerie contrast between the youthful vigor of dancing and the eternal stillness of death. The dances of death were part of a convivial attempt to deny the finality of death. Emphasizing the terrors of death, the dance was also an attempt to frighten sinners into repentance. Performers would beckon people to the hereafter in response to the Black Death.

Graves scarcely closed and the sight of sufferers overtook mourners and others with a strange morbid delusion and compulsion to perform in the churches or streets the dances of Saint John or Saint Vitus, their patron saints. Dancers formed a circle, hand in hand, and moved in wild delirium, howling, screaming, jumping, laughing involuntarily, until they fell to the ground in exhaustion. During the paroxysm, dancers were haunted by visions of spirits, blood, and the Virgin Mary.

Evolving with the skeletal figure seen as the future self, the dance not only mocked the pretenses of the rich who abused their positions on earth but also pointed to a vision of social equality. The death figure dances convulsively, lording it over mortals, who are sent a somber message.

After the harvest in certain years, hallucination, a sense of suffocation and burning, and cramp symptoms of ergot (a rye fungus) poisoning, called

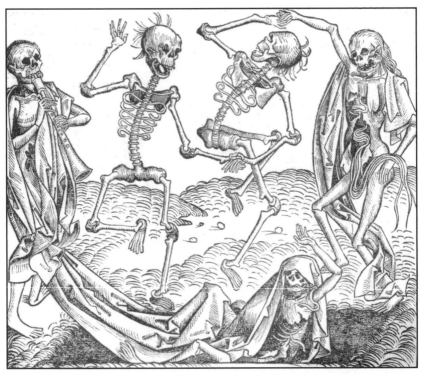

**Figure 4.1.** Dance of Death (from Schedel Hartmann, *Liber Cronicarum*, Nuremberg, 1493, p. 264. Courtesy of the Clendening History of Medicine Library, University of Kansas, Medical Center)

Saint Anthony's Fire, led some of the sickly victims to move involuntarily in dancelike movements. The dancing victims were believed to be possessed by invading demons. Other victims sought relief from pain through ecstatic dancing that matched the convulsive movements of Saint John's and Saint Vitus's dances, considered to be of curative value and likely to ward off death. Louis Backman, who identified the association between the symptoms and alkaloid poisoning from ergot, has concluded that dancing would indeed provide a symptomatic relief for the victims until the poison worked its way through their systems.[17] However, the mania for dance was more widespread than the poisoning. Dancing appears to have served key cathartic, working-through, and other stress-management functions.

Dancing was part of wakes for the dead, and the rebirth of the soul to everlasting life. At the graves of family, friends, and martyrs, dancing was believed to comfort the dead and encourage resurrection in addition to protecting them from the dead's manifestations as demons.

## Ketjak

The Balinese *ketjak* (called the Monkey Dance, although it concerns humans and only incidentally animals) was a traditional religious performance used during stressful times of peril and pestilence. *Ketjak* refers to the sounds voiced by a male chorus (in lieu of an orchestra) that accompany several kinds of dances intended both to stimulate trance states in individuals and to promote purification (*sangyang*) of a village. Phillip McKean[18] witnessed ceremonies that started in December and were performed nightly for four months and then every fifth night for another month. A local priest first prepared offerings and incense. The spirits then incarnated themselves in two young girls about fourteen years old. Bodily recipients of *dedari*, meaning heavenly nymphs, they would dance *Sangyang Dedari,* a dance believed to exorcise evil and bring a blessing. They danced well into the night before emerging from the trance. During this dancing, the *ketjak* dance itself began and lasted for several hours.

From purity to pollution? McKean asks. Since coming into contact with the West, the dance has also become a popular tourist attraction in which the

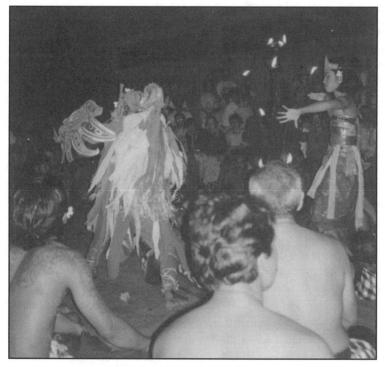

**Figure 4.2.** *Ketjak* **(Photo by Judith Lynne Hanna)**

sacred and profane coexist. For economic gain, Balinese now perform *ketjak* in tourist hotels. This performance, however, is different in its condensation, selective sharing, and meaning for the participants. Limited to an hour, much of the traditional ceremony is consequently omitted. Yet the Balinese retain their religious obligations that follow from devotion to a hierarchy of gods, demons, spirits, and wraiths, which they acknowledge to have power or control over their lives. Moreover, there seems to remain an intuitive meaning, a peculiar way of seeing, in the *ketjak* that is not vitiated by the commercial enterprise of tourist entertainment.

## Shakers

Dance in its kaleidoscopic variety is sometimes a means to manage the stress of a repressed sex drive. Sexual energy is channeled into dance in which the performer sublimates sexual consummation. A remarkable example is found among the United Society of Believers in Christ's Second Appearing, commonly called the Shakers because of their dramatic practice of vigorous dancing to crush sexual desire and dispel sin. Consisting of about six thousand members in nineteen communities at its peak in the United States, the group believed that the day of judgment was imminent and that salvation would come through confessing and forsaking fleshly practices. Sexual conduct became a benchmark of an individual's morality and the basis for reward or punishment in the next life. The Shakers believed that if lust were conquered, other problems would solve themselves.

Ann Lee (1736–1784), a founder of this utopian millenary society, had experiences that played a central role in shaping Shaker theology and practice.[19] Lee had deep feelings of guilt and shame about her strong sex drive, a sense of impurity concerning the fleshly cohabitation of the sexes, and a prurient interest in the sex lives of others. Her turbulent marriage led to eight bitter and harrowingly difficult pregnancies. Lee's offspring were stillborn or died in early childhood, only one living to six years. Sexual coition had caused her suffering. During one of her periods of imprisonment (the Shakers were frequently persecuted), she received a revelation of Adam and Eve's first "carnal act," which she interpreted as the source of human depravity. She then promulgated a revulsion toward sexuality. Lee was concerned with the plight of women in marriage, which she likened to servitude; prostitution; rape; and the risks of pregnancy and parturition. Women's bodies were maimed through men's primitive knowledge of their bodily functions.[20] The Shakers thus saw woman as a victim abused by irresponsible men for their selfish pleasure.

Choosing celibacy, Lee became a universal mother and sublimated her sex drive in spiritualization. "She called herself, and was considered by her followers, the 'Second Appearing of Christ'. . . As a female Christ she stood in the place of spiritual mate to the male Christ. She is reputed to have told the Elders on one occasion that Christ 'is my Lord and Lover' (a spiritual lover impregnating her with the lives of regenerated souls)."[21] A female image of God did empower women in the Shaker community. Their social organization was based on the equality of the sexes and emphasized group rather than individual pursuits.

Notwithstanding Shaker attitudes toward transcending the body through sheer willpower, the first adherents were seized by an involuntary and repressed passion. It led them to run about a meeting room, jump, hop, tremble, whirl, reel in a spontaneous manner, and wrestle with the Devil to shake off the flesh and doubts, loosen sins and faults, induce humility, and purge the body of lust in order to purify the spirit. In their pursuit of repentance they turned away from preoccupation with self to shake off their bondage to a troubled past in a febrile performance called "laboring." The attempt to escape the body while being riveted to it permitted concentration on new feelings and intent.

In this release of energy mobilized in the stress response and working through, individualistic impulsive and ecstatic abandon eventually evolved into ordered, well-rehearsed, drill-like group dance-movement patterns over the two hundred years of the sect's existence. Shaking the hand palm

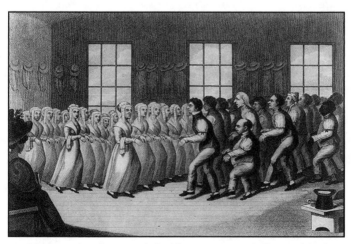

**Figure 4.3. Shakers Diverting Sexual Sin (Photo courtesy of Library of Congress, Prints and Photographs Division)**

downward discarded the carnal; turning palms upward petitioned eternal life. The square, circle, line or march, and endless change, comprised the spatial design. Herein male and female often came in proximity to each other, yet they never touched. The shaking-off-sin movement sequence parallels the sexual experience of energy build-up to climax and then relaxation. Both sexes dancing conveyed images of a process of the pursuit of purity and denial of sexuality.[22]

For the Shakers, who believed in the dualism of spirit versus body, their dancing appeared to be a channeling of feeling in the context of men and women living together in celibacy, austerity, humility, and hard manual labor. Dancing afforded an outlet for energies restrained by Shaker regimentation, and a sanctioned emotional release from the enforced separation of the sexes. Men and women were apart except for during the worship service, of which dance was a central part, and the rare "union" or visiting meetings.

## Afterword

Tarantism, dances of death, *ketjak*, and Shakerism encompass religious world-views about physical phenomena and supernatural power. These dances were ways of coping with a host of stresses: puberty crises; sexual frustration; spider bites; plagues; ergot poisoning; economic, female, and political exploitation; and need for attention. The participants engaged in both autogenic and directive styles of dealing with stress. In their attempts to reduce stress, their dancing was psychologically and physically cathartic and provided avenues for altered states of consciousness. For the most part, the purposes of the dances were not explicitly articulated. Moreover, dance provided pretexts for behavior that would not otherwise be acceptable or possible. The Shakers, however, in their extreme view of sexuality, were clear about the movement of shaking off sin and sublimating sexual passion in a sanctioned release. Dance released the energy generated in the stress response that mobilized the body to repress the sex drive. A means to manage anxiety and fear, dance required the creation of supportive social networks and symbolic enactments of problems and desired actions.

~

## CHAPTER FIVE

# Coming to Terms with Life Crises

## Marriage, Life, and Death in Ubakala Igbo Dance-Plays

Although Nigeria's Ubakala Igbo dance-plays could be taken as representative of Africa, bear in mind that the continent has about one thousand different language groups, and probably that many different dance-pattern constellations. A group usually has many different kinds of dances and participation criteria.[1]

Ubakala dance-plays are conceived, produced, performed, and responded to in terms of an interweaving of the intrinsic characteristics of the dance-play genre and the extrinsic characteristics of Ubakala culture and society. From my 1963 fieldwork in Africa, I have found the dance-plays to be an expression of emotion or its symbolization, as well as an expression of ideas.[2] As such, the dance-play appears to be a psychotherapeutic vehicle for the diagnosis, prevention, and treatment of stress-related personal and social disorders. The dance-play serves as catharsis, anticipatory psychic management, illness prevention, and paradox mediation (discussed in chapter 6).

A few basic contextual facts are relevant to understanding how the dance-play helps people cope with potentially stressful life crises. The Ubakala are one of about two hundred formerly politically autonomous Igbo groups in Nigeria. In terms of social organization, descent is traced on the father's side, and a married couple and their children live with the father's family. There is a sexually based division of agricultural labor, in part biologically determined on the basis of reproductive and physical-strength capabilities. Reincarnation and ancestor honor are key tenets in the traditional polytheistic religion, which persists to some degree even among converted Christians. Traditionalists may add Jesus to their pantheon of deities and spirits.

The dance-play (nkwa) among the Ubakala appears to approximate the human-potential, or self-actualization, model of dance therapy and the preventive-medicine, or wellness, model rather than the medical model. Ubakala dance-plays help to maintain cultural patterns and provide stability for individuals; that is, norms for social life are presented in the performances. The dance-play is a method of indoctrination about the individual's role, sense of self-worth, and group support. Through the nkwa, individuals have a medium to assist them in achieving their fullest potential, adapting to the social environment, and changing distasteful aspects of the social milieu. The dance-play reflects, influences, and is part of many other aspects of the society and culture in which it is embedded. Dance may be viewed as a language of command and control, that is, a vehicle of power that gives the dancer the ability to influence others' predispositions, feelings, attitudes, beliefs, and actions.

Specific mechanisms of dance-play "group therapy" focus on preventing stress by engaging participants in anticipatory psychic management of life crises and alternative catharsis.[3] A method of socialization, anticipatory psychic management prepares an individual for a threatening experience by rehearsing it until its potential destructive emotional impact is reduced to manageable proportions. Systematic desensitization[4] is the equivalent term in behavior modification. "Every fresh repetition," wrote Freud, "seems to strengthen this mastery for which [the individual] strives."[5] The therapeutic efficacy is not in sheer repetition but in "active reproduction or recreation and . . . transformation through various mechanisms, characteristic of artistic production."[6]

Usually, repetition in order to manage or assimilate a situation or feeling relates to a past traumatic event. However, repetition can also help manage anticipated future events. Among the Ubakala, anticipatory psychic management appears to be most commonly associated with the tensions of adulthood, for example, getting married, giving birth, and coping with death. Typical of the anticipation of womanhood is the Nkwa Edere (young girls' shimmy dance-play). In several of the specific dances, the movement refers to anxieties and emotional occasions in the life of an adult woman, namely, heterosexual relations, becoming a wife and leaving one's natal home, being fertile, and giving birth. Young girls within the age of puberty (eleven to sixteen years old) focus on the hazards they will most likely face as they pass into adulthood.

The dance Ogbede Turuime (pregnant child) refers to a small girl's fear that when she marries she may be infertile and when she becomes pregnant

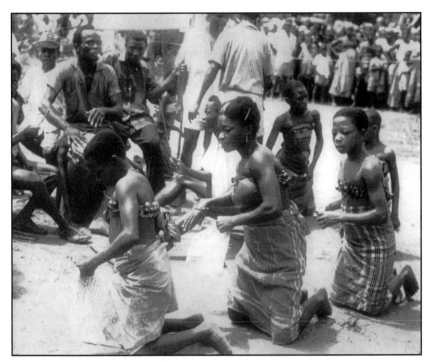

**Figure 5.1. Anticipating Marriage and Childbirth (Photo of Ubakala by William John Hanna)**

she might not deliver successfully (without modern medical treatment, childbirth is a dangerous process during which tragedy may occur for seemingly inexplicable reasons). A broader concern is the transition from childhood to adulthood. This transition is more traumatic for a girl than for a boy because for her, marriage means leaving the familiar home environment to live among strangers—her husband and his kin (among whom she is not fully accepted as a family member)—and at the same time adjusting to her new roles of wife and mother. "Being a wife . . . is no easy matter."[7] In fact, young brides are known to run away to their birthplace from home sickness and other distress. Yet at the separation of a bride from her ancestral lineage, elderly women console the girl and her mother by reminding them that what is involved is a journey and not death.

In *Nkwa Edere*, the shoulders shimmy in many of the dance movements as the pelvis shifts from side to side. Breast development and other pubescent body changes are thus highlighted. Girls create different dance movement sequences to show their creativity and physical endurance, characteristics men seek in a wife. The girls dance a one-two-three-hold conga pattern, moving counterclockwise in a circle; they creatively reverse directions on the hold. Then they dance the conga sequence on their knees. All the while the torso is forward-inclined as if the dancer is entreating the beneficence of the fruit-giving earth deity for human fertility.

Aspects of both the *Nkwa Uko* (dance-play for the death of an elderly woman) and the *Nkwa Ese* (dance-play for the death of an elderly man) also appear to be anticipatory psychic management, because they familiarize participants with the rituals accompanying death, reminding them of the coming of their own deaths and their opportunity to eventually achieve ancestor status.[8] The *Nkwa Uko* dance titled "The Deceased Are Blessed" suggests this.

These dance-plays for the deceased appear to release the living from the stresses imposed by death in a way that is minimally disruptive, to give the living an opportunity to anticipate and thus better manage their lives in regard to their own demise, and to communicate the clan's beliefs about life and death. Second burials (rituals to assist the buried deceased in her or his journey to the ancestor world) and other mourning ceremonies constitute institutionalized means of gradually working through the loss. If all affect were discharged at once, the result could be overwhelming individual stress and group disruption. The communal solidarity experienced in the *nkwa* and the physical expenditure of tension in its performance help to improve group morale and dissipate anxiety; it is a psychological support for members of the bereaved family, for whom death has disturbed existing social and ritual relationships and of whom adjustment is demanded. Thus the dance-plays appear to provide a useful vehicle for tension release and prevention of stress.

Despite the universality of death, its rationalization, and the Ubakala belief that ancestors are the continuation of a lineage's living representatives, considerable anxiety about death still exists.[9] The first reactions to death for the Igbo are disgust, annoyance, pain, and a sense of loss, for death is indiscriminate in killing good and wicked alike.[10] "This anxiety is often well hidden in formalized ways of talking about illness, or in cure-seeking rituals . . . every blessing, be it of the ancestors in the serving of palm wine, be that a sacrifice, contains the statement, 'Let there be long life.'"[11]

In the *Nkwa Ese* dance-play for a deceased man, dancing out anger in response to death is a form of symbolic concretization. It involves the transformation of a wish, thought, or mood into a mock interpersonal encounter. The dance-play externally fixes and codifies feelings that may have been repressed or concealed.

Through machete- and stick-brandishing advances and retreats, the male dancers in the *Nkwa Ese* vigorously portray as warriorlike the deeds, exploits,

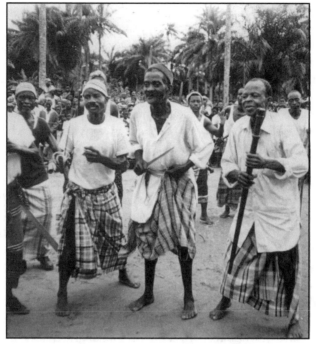

**Figure 5.2.   Men (Photo of Ubakala by William John Hanna)**

and prowess of the deceased or his ancestors in order to bestow praise and honor upon him and his descendants. In the *Nkwa Uko* the women dance in much the same way as they do for the celebration of the birth of a child. However, physical contact occurs occasionally when two women, each with an arm around the other's waist, dance together at the center of the circle, as a sign of condolence.

In a society whose members' religious beliefs include reincarnation, participating in a ceremony concerning the death of another may give individuals an opportunity to cope more effectively with the stresses associated with the coming of their own deaths. This coping mechanism is most evident when the ceremony emphasizes generational continuity and praises the dead.

Catharsis, another dance-play group-therapy mechanism used to prevent stress, is experienced through enervating movements and/or transgressive criticism. The movements of Ubakala girls' and women's dance-plays appear to provide outlets for females' fears about the uncertainties of a successful birth, sanctions for failure, and pain related to marriage and childbirth. Similarly the dance-plays for the deceased provide outlets for the emotional stress that accompanies the loss of a loved one and fear of the deceased's spirit.

A newborn child represents a triumph over the odds of infant mortality. Large families are necessary for agricultural work, protection, and security in old age and provide a manpower reservoir capable of replacing the victims of infant mortality, war, and disease to ensure perpetuation of the group. Having offspring marks success in life. Children must perform the dance-play to ensure the deceased's journey to the world of the ancestors, from which rebirth occurs in the form of the birth of a grandchild or other incarnation. Death is seen as merely the terminus of one phase of time and space. "For a person to die without children to perform funeral rituals for him is a tragedy. Implicitly it means, of course, that he is soon likely to be forgotten, for who will sacrifice to him as an ancestor?"[12] Who will "offer . . . the daily prayers, libations of wine, and sacrifices of kola nuts or pieces of food?"[13] Having many surviving children brings a parent prestige and marks success in life. Indeed, an Ubakala woman's marriage and personal status depend on this.

Yet childbirth has its hazards. The dance-play performed to rejoice for the birth of a child appears to provide a safety-valve mechanism for the release of women's delivery tension, pain, and anxiety about infant mortality—emotions that might otherwise be directed toward dysfunctional activities. In deference to the pregnant women participating, the dance tempo is slow, and the movement texture sustained; however, anxiety may be reduced through continuous motion, full-throated song, and explosive yells and ululations. Perhaps as compensation for being considered the inferior sex in a male-dominated society, this vivid dance-play, which proclaims the great achievement of women, is a means of female self-assertion.

Dance is often restorative in allowing an individual to reassert the impulsive after the strain of adapting and the weariness of conforming. Deviant movement patterns, a form of catharsis, occur in the *Nkwa Edere* waltz dance. In pairs, the girls embrace and caress each other as they dance. The embracing European ballroom dance position is a parody of male-female behavior, which is not traditionally approved of (but occurs in urban areas). Public displays of physical contact between men and women are not seen in Ubakala villages. Safier writes: "Convention dictates which postures, stance, carriage or gait we assume in this or that area of life. Dance is perceived as an escape from this restraint although dance brings with it is own bondage in the stylization of movement. At least dance movements are different from the movements of routine living. Thus dance encourages relaxation in both reality and in illusion."[14]

Transgressive criticism through the dance-play, which serves as a legitimate vehicle for otherwise prohibited or inappropriate social commentary and criticism, joking, or aggression, may be cathartic. Donatus Ibe Nwoga argues that the salutary purpose of satire is incidental to the "idea of punishment through words. It is anger with a person or a group, rather than the sense of offended morality, which is the principal urge."[15]

## Samburu Role Transition and Dance

Another case of catharsis and coming to terms with life-cycle crises comes from northern Kenya. Here, the Samburu dances are both markers and outlets for stresses related to passage from one phase of the life cycle to another. Boys of about fourteen years of age eagerly look forward to initiation into warriorhood, the privileges of which, including close association with girls, are jealously guarded by the existing *moran*, or warrior age set. The age set of *moran* retires to elderhood at about thirty years of age, marrying and settling down when the next age set takes over. There is an implicit element of coercion when the boys unite in dance to demand circumcision, because it legitimates them as a new set of future warriors. The assertiveness of the boys' circumcision dance expresses their restlessness and anticipation of circumcision.

The dances of the *moran*, who are prohibited from marrying in an order imposed by the elders, seem to be a temporary release of the built-up tension that is associated with a young person's restricted position in society.[16] The Samburu's flexible nomadic existence makes a monogamous family too small to be economically viable as an independent unit. Consequently, the Samburu have developed a social organization structured by polygyny, a delayed marriage age for men, and leadership by mature adult men, who monopolize formal power and nubile women. In the interim, a *moran* can have a young adolescent mistress within his clan, although he cannot marry her. Older women are married and involved in homemaking activities.

There is a concerted force manifest in a suppressed sector of Samburu society. "The *moran* and girls [who join them in special dances] do not merely release tension, but they also develop a camaraderie, united through the dance in a token protest against the regime under which they are placed."[17] The dancing provides a gauge of sentiment that the elders cannot ignore when they see the dance reigning supreme with its alternative undomesticated order.

In preparation for a dance, the *moran* carefully adorn themselves with their loin cloths and paint glistening red ocher on their faces and shoulders. They try to outdo each other in self-display and boasting in the dance. At first the *moran* usually dance *nbarinkoi*. In a tight chanting group, they rhythmically move forward together, "twice raising their heels, bending their knees, thrusting their heads forwards and exhaling audibly—in fact not unlike bulls—and then straightening themselves and lifting their spears on the third beat."[18]

Then comes *nkokorri* dancing. It incorporates provocative thrusting movements with assertive bull-like grunting, followed by jumping movements as the dancers rise and fall in unison. The dance climaxes with shivering movements. A display of manliness and the urge to fight, as well as an act that makes a man irresistible in battle, the quivering accompanies a "tightness gripping their chests, inducing a sense of breathless suffocation as they sink into unconsciousness and achieve relaxation."[19] The girls, who have also carefully adorned themselves for the occasion of the dance, look on. After these two male dances of display, the girls as a group join in the dance. Taunting the youths to engage in cattle rustling, the girls partake in vicarious rebelliousness.

The elders control the marriages of their daughters to men in another clan, where they will start a new life in a position of complete subservience. The claims of the *moran* over these girls as lovers are overridden. Each wedding sharply reminds all *moran* and girls of the elders' power to interfere in their affairs. Consequently, a wedding is "the principal occasion at which *moran* are popularly expected to express their protest in a display of anger through dancing."[20] The dance is one of the opposed forces of assertiveness and constraint. Very angry *moran* may "break down in an insensible fit of convulsive shaking" in response to the paradoxical stress.[21] At successful dances, as many as five or more *moran* will break down in this way, following each other in relatively quick succession. And then after the trembling subsides and they regain their composure, they return to the dance, apparently cured of their bout of anger as they merge almost passively into the main body of dancers. Energy mobilized by the stress response is released in the dance.

Married men do not dance. However, married women have their dances for fertility, which provide a measure of temporary escape from domestic chores and male dominance.

## Lugbara Dances for Death and Life's Uncertainty

Through their dancing, the Lugbara of Uganda convey messages about their desire for a stable society; the social and cosmic relations in which they are involved are always uncertain and beyond their comprehension. Yet the dance is one means by which they try to comprehend and resolve the stress of structural ambiguity.[22]

Anticipatory psychic management is operative in dances related to death. The Lugbara, like the Ubakala, mark the process of change from living to dead in rites of transition. "At death the constituent elements of the person separate and move from the social sphere to those beyond it. The soul goes to divinity in the sky, the spirit to the wilderness . . . the soul is later re-domesticated by diviners and the spirit remains in the bush land. During this process the social status of the deceased is uncertain, beyond contact by the living, who cannot enter into any direct relationship with him or her: after the establishment of a shrine they may do so again."[23]

Integral to Lugbara mortuary rites are two dances. Wailing dances, *ongo* or *auwu-ongo*, take place soon after a death, sometimes even prior to the actual burial. They show respect to the deceased, who would otherwise be insulted and possibly send sickness or nightmares to his or her living kin or appear to them as a specter. Playing dances (*abi* or *avico-ongo*) are performed a year after a death. Lineage members of the deceased dance and wail, whereas affines "play" to express the joy that reaffirms kinship ties after the lineage is disrupted. The order of dancing, with each group praising the prowess of its own lineage segments and attacking the others, conveys the constellation of lineage ties that has been disrupted by death. The death dance for an important man may attract well over a hundred people, some of whom become drunk and aggressive.

A special feature of the dance is a trancelike condition that occurs after a long period of performing and drinking on a relatively empty stomach. The resulting inadequate blood flow to the brain causes dizziness and other altered states of consciousness. These may link the dancers as distinct individuals to the soul of the deceased, in a dramatic retreat from customary relations with others within the lineage group. The opiumlike pain-killing chemicals released in the dance may help to heal the stress of death.

The dance participants are primarily men, who dance as a group. In two lines set within a circle of onlookers, the men leap up and down in inward concentration with legs straight and together, arms either stretched out above the head or holding weapons symbolic of masculinity. Women, in contrast, dance individually or as groups of sisters; they hop loosely and hold their arms out in front of them at shoulder level, bent at the elbow in a supple waving gesture.

Certain women's dances bear a resemblance to death dances in that they are performed when there is uncertainty. For example, women dance *nyambi* as an intervention for anxiety immediately after a delayed harvest due to excessive rain or at the end of a long dry season. During these irregular times, intergroup quarreling and fighting over scarce resources are common. The women dance to the area where the rainmaker awaits them and then performs rites to reset the disorderly passing of time and repair disorderly social relations. Seemingly a mirror reflection of the death dance in which men dance in lines of patrilineal kin, women of the subclan dance together irrespective of lineage and affinal affiliations.

## Death/Disorder to Life/Order

I have described some stress-management approaches that occur in dance rituals of transformation. At life crises, these performances permit individuals to anticipate future crises as well as accept them in a positive vein through catharsis. In Tanzania, the Nyakyusa's funeral dance begins with a passionate expression of anger and grief and gradually becomes a fertility dance. In this way dancing mediates the passionate and quarrelsome emotions felt over a death and the acceptance of it, the uncontrolled and controlled.[24]

Among the Dogon of Mali, death creates a special kind of disorder. Yet through the masked dance, humans metaphorically restore order to the

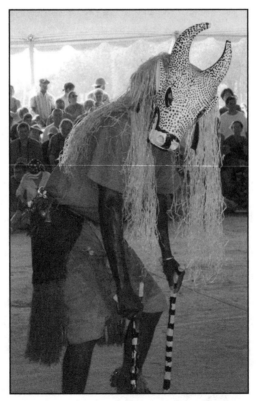

**Figure 5.3.   Ordering the Disordered (Photo of Dogon by Judith Lynne Hanna)**

stressful world in a like-equals-reality conception. Symbolizing in space a world they have not seen, the Dogon illustrate the representation of heaven on earth. Their cosmic image is conventionally reflected in the arrangement of villages in pairs, one representing heaven, the other earth, and in their fields, which are cleared spirally, as the world is believed to have been created. So, too, at the time of death, masked dancers represent all aspects of Dogon life. Masked dancers drive out the spirits that might bring chaos. The spirits of the dead return to the afterworld to rest and leave the village free from disruption. Some dancers representing "beings of the bush," everything that is wild and beyond man's control, also perform in order to help the community deal with the psychic distress and spiritual fear of the dead. Order exists in the dancing in its specific symbolism and patterns in the spheres of the funerary event, the total human body (which is conceived of as an image of the cosmos) in action, the organic and discursive performance, specific movements, and other forms of communication, particularly costume.[25]

## Afterword

We have seen how the dance medium is a vehicle through which people come to terms with the hallmarks of life—birth, sexual drive, marriage, ecological harm, social disorder, death, and uncertainty. The rituals—through anticipation, catharsis, group protest, altered states of consciousness, and symbolic enactment—allow people to resist stress, reduce it when it occurs, or temporarily escape it. The stress intervention style is autogenic, although cultural traditions are directive in providing expectations for the dance performance. Recall that when you neither fight nor flee from stress because physical action in the immediate situation is uncalled for, biochemical elements of energy may remain in the body and cause harm. Dancing absorbs this energy.

∽

## CHAPTER SIX

# Resolving Conflict

In this chapter, I describe two cases of secular social/ethnic dance that I observed during my fieldwork in Africa in the 1960s and in the United States in the 1970s. The first focuses on the Ubakala Igbo's use of dance in social drama in Nigeria, and the second centers on African American play with dance in a desegregated school in Dallas. These cases that illustrate how dance is a communicative medium with the ability to move people to consider ideas and actions for resolving stressful situations.

Central to these cases is the concept of dance as play—a safe arena for exploring beyond the known or working through problems, an exercise of mental or physical faculties, and an activity for survival. Play maintains a "regular, crisis-oriented expenditure of kinetic energy" that can be "switched from play-energy into fight-energy."[1]

## Ubakala Social Drama

A mode of communication, the dance-play engages an individual with potentially stressful concerns in a communal activity with persons close to her or him. As in family and community therapy,[2] the dance-play makes public stressful grievances for conflict resolution. Because some of the Ubakala's values are contradictory, and the pursuit of one to the exclusion of the other creates a paradox, the dance-play becomes a diagnostic tool through its presentation of the issues, and a mediator through the catalyst of remedial action.

Paradox mediation, a form of stress prevention and remediation, refers to the resolution of conflicting opposites. Fundamental and sometimes conflicting, Ubakala values move people to social action. An emphasis on individual competition and achievement is juxtaposed with the need for co-operation and interdependence (community spirit, group solidarity, and shar-ing the wealth; personal aggrandizement is not emphasized). The desire for and expectation of change often run counter to the principle of respect for authority; this is largely based on seniority. Innovation generally involves criticism or rejection of what those older than oneself have established. The principle of respect and obedience to leaders is opposed both to the egalitar-ian distaste for assertive authority and to the norm of bringing things into the open.

If an individual or group pursues one part of a pair of opposites to the exclusion of the other, this creates an imbalance, dilemma, and social drama. When one value is expressed such that it violates another equally valid value, and an individual or group feels threatened and desires to contain, modify, or reverse it, the dance-play is able to mediate between persons and their situations (in much the same way as speech mediates between persons and their situations or a shaman mediates unbalanced forces in a healing ritual). The dance-play has the potential to mediate social relations and political situations by encapsulating the issues and phases of social dramas. The four phases of social drama are (1) a breach of the norms of a social group, (2) a mounting crisis, (3) a legal or ritual process of remediation, and (4) public and symbolic expression of an irreparable schism or reconciliation.[3] Accordingly, the dance-play may communicate a breach, foment a crisis, ameliorate the conflict (or at least hold it in suspension so that it is present, viewable, and worth considering), and proclaim the schism or celebrate the reintegration.

The Ubakala allow a special kind of license in the dance-play that protects the individual and group from libel and allows alternative social arrangements to be played with, exciting programs to be undermined, and new ones to be generated. Contrary ways of acting and thinking, perhaps ultimately unwork-able or having disastrous consequences, or normative ways with a positive impact may be presented. The dance-play is a vehicle for negotiating sepa-rate personalities, individual biographies, into a shared entity to transform personal experience and thus create a certain degree of anonymity.

The dance-play has the potential for more than letting off the steam of energy mobilized in the stress response or catharsis: It can guard against the misuse of power and produce social change without violence. However, the messages of dance-plays are often implicit; and a symbolic system is a weak vehicle of control unless enforcement follows. The dance-play is a political form of coercion in a shame-oriented society. Energy (force), the ultimate means of social control, is symbolically represented.

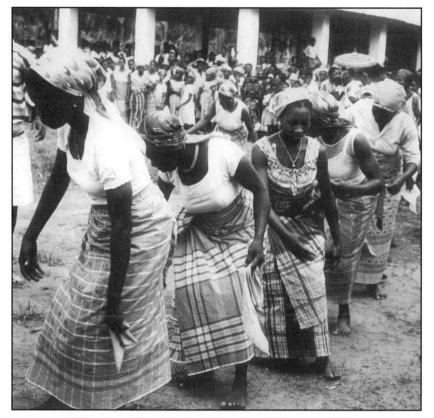

**Figure 6.1.** Women (Photo of Ubakala by William John Hanna)

An illustration of the use of the dance-play to prevent and reduce stress is the Ubakala "outsider" society dance-play. Biologically related women who have married into the same village organize as an expression of unity to counter the bonds of blood and kin that bind their husbands. Living as they do among "strangers," and having little part in formal political and religious activities, women who hail from the same natal village seek each other out. Their goals are to rejoice in the fact that they have children, to confront jointly the problems of family life, to share economic resources, and to affirm friendships among their kindred. These women especially use the dance-play to adjust wrongdoings and work through the contradictions of social life and so reduce stress.

The famous 1929 "women's war" in which the dance-play communication went unheeded illustrates the power of this women's medium. Repercussions were widespread on both local and intercontinental levels. Contemporary politicians and leaders refer to this notorious episode of feminine protest as reason to consider women's views.[4] They remember how the women moved the British to alter their colonial administration of eastern Nigeria.

Women's intrusion into the affairs of state, and their imposition of sanctions, makes them the custodians of the "constitution," the basic governing principles of Ubakala society.[5] Because women marry outside the village group into which they were born, their kin organization cuts across and goes beyond any one level of political structure. The organization is thus powerful in its ability to rally numerous groupings behind any single member.

When performed as a boycott, the women's dance-play is sometimes called "sitting on a man."[6] The aggrieved gather at the compound of an offender and dance and sing to detail the problem. Movement presents a dynamic image emphasizing the argument as well as releasing and generating physical and psychological energy and tension. The accompanying song, with its potent ridicule and satire, serves as a vehicle for specific social criticism.

The British colonial government of Nigeria was generally aware of the potential for public disturbance catalyzed through this cultural expression. Thus its native council was empowered in 1901 to regulate "native plays [gatherings] . . . of natives in any public street or market, or in any house, building, or in any compound adjoining a public street or market for the purpose of dancing or playing native music."[7] In some areas, licenses and permission from the British district commissioner were necessary to hold plays.

A breach of understanding between women and the colonial government heralded the first phase of the social drama. In 1928 the British government introduced taxation, which was applicable only to men. Late in 1929, women incorrectly believed that this tax was to be extended to them. This misunderstanding signaled the beginning of an example of "sex solidarity and political power which women can exercise when they choose to do so."[8]

The women viewed taxation as an infringement upon their economic competitive patterns. In the latter part of the nineteenth century, women started to amass considerable wealth from cultivating and trading in palm kernels. Not appreciating the economic and political position of women, the British attempted to focus hitherto-diffuse power on Nigerian male warrant chiefs appointed by the colonial government. Since women had not become representatives of the colonial government as Nigerian men had, the women did not see how they would benefit from the imposition of taxes. The women's economic and political grievances coalesced. Women were aggrieved by the European control of market prices, and what they considered the abusive and extortionist practices of many colonial government-appointed Nigerian warrant chiefs (for example, some obtained wives without paying full bride wealth; others took property inappropriately).

Nigerians were in the midst of a an economic depression, the effects of which hurt women, when a young British assistant district officer in Bende Division ignited the conflagration. Because census registers were incomplete and inaccurate, the administrative officers were supposed to revise the initial counts in their spare time. In October, Captain John Cook (who had taken over from A. L. Weir, who had deceived the people in 1927 about the purpose of the initial tax census) decided on his own authority to obtain information from the warrant chief about the number of men, women, children, and livestock in the district.

A massive protest broke out when the Warrant Chief Okugo of Oloko Village, near the town of Aba, employed a school teacher, Mark Emeruwa, to take charge of the census. Inquiring about the possessions of a local woman, Nwanyeruwa, he engaged in an argument and physical scuffle with her. Fearing further deprivations by the colonialists, she then reported the incident to her village women's meeting.

As women gathered to discuss what had occurred, a mounting crisis marked the second phase of the social drama. The alarmed women sent palm leaves, symbols of warning and distress, to the women of neighboring and distant villages, summoning them to Okoko to join the protest. Women from far and near, even pregnant women, met in Okoko's square on November 24.

The third stage of the social drama was the potentially remedial process of sitting on a man, which usually works to resolve conflicts and ward off stress. (The audience-captivating dance-play medium serves as a socially acceptable vehicle to express strong displeasure, which in turn has the effect of catalyzing people to act to ameliorate the cause of dissatisfaction.) The irate women trooped to the mission that employed Emeruwa, the chief's messenger, to demonstrate against him. They camped in front of his compound at the Niger Delta Mission and "sat on him," meaning the man was kept from sleeping and carrying out his usual tasks. The women danced and sang outside the mission compound all night, eating, drinking palm wine, and singing that Nwanyeruwa had been told to count her goats, sheep, and people.[9] A song was quickly improvised to meet the situation. The women sent their message. Yet no satisfactory response was forthcoming.

The next day, with the problem still unresolved, the social drama reached the schism phase. The women became more excited and went to the chief's compound. They besieged Chief Okugo at his house and demanded his cap of office, a symbol of his authority. He escaped to seek refuge at the Native Court compound. Captain Cook met with over 25,000 women in the market to assure them they were not to be taxed; however, the women insisted that Chief Okugo and Emeruwa be arrested and tried.

Skeptical of government assurances that they were not to be taxed, the women's rampages continued. Late in December, the women forced the Umuahia town warrant chiefs to surrender their caps. In the town of Aba, women sang and danced to no avail about their antipathy toward the chiefs and the court messengers. So they proceeded to attack and loot the European trading stores and Barclays Bank and to break into the prison and release its prisoners.[10]

The riots spread, involving about 10,000 women in two provinces. Destruction was directed primarily toward the warrant chiefs and buildings representing this detested authority. Finally, in panic, the British authorities called troops and police into the area. A car accident and heated passions triggered the most extreme violence. In the town of Opobo in Calabar Province, the police opened fire in one of the worst episodes; thirty-two women were killed, and thirty-one wounded.[11] News of the slaughter spread, and local disturbances persisted well into 1930.

The women's rapid mobilization was possible because of their strong societal organization and effective communication networks based on their association in the markets and along the trade routes. Colonial government reorganizations in 1930–1931 followed the recommendations of two commissions of inquiry and anthropological studies. The women succeeded in the destruction of warrant chief system. The cost and stress would have been less had the audience (i.e., the government) been more attentive initially to the dance-play. Thus the contemporary women's performance serves as a metaphor for their power.[12]

Linked to the memories or stories of dramatic instances of unheeded dance-plays is the dynamic concept of play, which may help to explain the role of the dance-play in conflict management. Play, as mentioned earlier, can maintain a pattern of kinetic energy, and people can draw upon this in a crisis situation.

## Race Relations in Dallas

The expression of grievances through dance to deal with stressful situations is widespread in Africa and the diaspora. Moreover, the arts, as a medium to critique society, are found worldwide. Therefore it is not surprising to find African American children dancing out their reactions to stressful events and ongoing social exchanges.

Needless to say, slavery and its aftermath have been difficult for blacks in the new world. Even desegregation, intended by public-policy makers to be helpful to blacks, was a source of anxiety. Let me share with you some of my observations from a year-long study of Pacesetter, an elementary school in Dallas.[13] At the time of my study, Pacesetter was newly desegregated with a court-ordered fifty-fifty black-white ratio in each classroom. Because of its superior program, this magnate school, which was located in a black neighborhood, attracted white families, mine included, whose children were bused to the school.

I probably would have dismissed the black children's spontaneous dancing I observed over the course of the year as merely play, as did the school staff, had it not been for my experience in Africa, where I discovered that dance both reflects and influences people's lives. Individuals dance their ethnic identity in the same way that their dress or military emblems announced who they were. Old and young alike use the medium of dance to comment on contemporary problems and solutions. So, what was going on at Pacesetter when children spontaneously danced?

Anthropologists look at the context of activities they seek to understand. So we do not view children's own dancing in school in isolation from the values and experiences of the communities that feed the schools. We also look to the past to help explain creative behavior, which may exist for its own sake or may be a defensive reaction and a means to cope with stress.

Historically, blacks in Dallas were forced to live in segregated areas and were often permitted some self-governance. Then, when whites realized the value of areas inhabited by blacks for roads, airports, and white residences, or when blacks began living too close to them, whites pushed the blacks out. Verbal intimidation, water-well destruction, bombings, and rezoning laws encouraged black relocation.

Pacesetter is located in a black community that was created in the 1950s as a result of the firebombing of black homes that had been purchased or were being built in formerly all-white residential areas—there were nine unsolved explosions in 1951! At the time there was a housing shortage. The black population in Dallas had increased from about 50,000 in 1940 to about 80,000 in 1950, and the housing shortage left 8,000 families in need of housing. Through the efforts of civic leaders in the Dallas Citizens Interracial Association, a segregated-housing project was undertaken within the city limits so that government regulatory services could be provided. The new community of one-story frame houses had its own shopping center, churches, and school.

However, desegregation changed the racial orientation and control of the school. A five-year U.S. Justice Department effort culminated in 1975 when the presiding judge accepted a plan for whites to be bused on a voluntary basis to Pacesetter. The black community was originally middle class, so school and community leaders thought the cultural values of blacks and whites in the area would be similar. However, when laws were passed against segregated housing, many middle-income blacks moved into other more affluent neighborhoods, and lower-income blacks moved in.

At Pacesetter, desegregation brought together black and white students, neighborhood friendship groups and individual volunteers bused to the school who were strangers to each other and the black children, and low-income (mostly black) and middle-income (mostly white) youngsters. The majority of black children had been together since preschool. Like friendship groups elsewhere, they did not always readily accept strangers, even if the strangers were black.

The black community was not unanimously in favor of desegregation. Because black-white proximity in the past had led to harassment of blacks, there was understandable mistrust and anxiety. Desegregation was stressful because blacks feared mistreatment. The white students who came to Pacesetter, on the other hand, tended to come from civil rights–oriented families and invite interracial friendships. Yet many black children felt the white students who volunteered to attend the court-ordered desegregated magnet school were invading their turf.

Although black children born during the late 1960s and 1970s era of black power may not have been discriminated against, they learned that members of their families had been. Thus the children were sensitive to anything that could possibly be interpreted as racism. They were wary of the whites whom they believed to be taking over their school. It had had an all-black faculty during segregation. However, with desegregation there were only two black teachers out of a total of forty, and one black assistant teacher out of twenty (though there were both black and white co-principals and counselors).

An assumption of desegregation is that low-income blacks will want to emulate middle-class whites and pick up their academic achievement patterns. However, at Pacesetter (as in schools throughout the country), where students were two grade levels behind middle-class whites and blacks in academic achievement the majority of low-income black children did not highly value academic achievement and do what was required to earn high marks. Indeed, some devalued and belittled the work ethic and activities of formal schooling and tried to disrupt the efforts of those who attempted to succeed.

Because of limited employment opportunities for blacks, education did not have the same positive payoff as it did for whites. And in the face of limited opportunity, there has not often been strong family and community support for black children's academic success.

In spite of the low esteem for academic success some of the black children at Pacesetter had, they were still sensitive to public criticism of their inadequate school work. This led them to seek arenas in which they could dominate and gain recognition. If one has few material possessions and little power in the adult world, as is the case with oppressed minorities and children, the body and its use become especially important. Dance and football were arenas black youngsters selected for excelling at Pacesetter.

Because children learn that what they say with words can get them into trouble, they often use body language to express their frustrations, anxiety, and challenges to authority. Dance appears to be a type of communication that protects youngsters' defiant thoughts and actions from the negative sanctions of the teacher or other school authority. Purposefully ambiguous in her or his communication, the sender of the message reserves the prerogative to insist on a harmless interpretation rather than a provocative one. Three illustrations suggest how black children at Pacesetter used the dance to deal with the stresses of having white teachers and classmates in a society with a history of racial discrimination:

### Illustration 1

One day, before the teacher had established control of a second-grade class, several black children were dramatic in their misbehavior. They yelled out remarks; walked about the room; played with furniture pretending it was gymnastic, musical, or military equipment; and pushed, pulled, or hit others. A black boy tried to cut a white girl's blond hair. A black girl kept talking loudly. In response to the white teacher's question, "Would you like to go out?" the youngster got up from her chair and walked into the aisle where she stood, feet apart and knees bent. She brought her knees together and apart four times while crossing her hands together and apart in unison with her knees in what we call a Charleston step. Then she scurried back to her assigned seat and sat down. Moments later she skipped to the door, opened it, picked up a book that was lying outside, and ran back to her place. Then she stood upon the chair seat and performed what in ballet is called an arabesque. Standing on the ball of one foot, she lifted the other leg backward as high as she could, one arm held diagonally up and forward, the other diagonally down. From this position, she laughingly lost her balance and fell to the floor. The teacher picked her up and carried her out of the classroom. During the girl's performance, her peers gave her their undivided attention.

The girl's dance movements can be construed as dramatically defying the white teacher by acting inappropriately during a formal lesson. Breaking the rules of both the white-dominated school and of traditional ballet style, the child mocked the teacher. Mockery, of course, is a way to deal with stress. The girl left her assigned seat and walked into the aisle to perform a

Charleston movement—part of the repertoire of several black African groups and part of her African American ethnic identity. Then, again, out of the appropriate time and place for ballet, she performed an arabesque movement—part of the elitist, white ethnic ballet tradition. To add a further incongruity, the child performed a dance movement usually danced on a stage or dance studio floor on the seat of a classroom chair. Feet were placed where the buttocks are supposed to be. Breaking these rules, the child sassed the teacher in a display of insubordination. Her deliberately clumsy fall, as she performed a movement that traditionally requires the dancer to assume a basic pose and then change the body support on one leg with elegant and graceful body control, was more than mere clownlike action.

The performance suggests once again the historical pattern of blacks parodying white behavior.[14] symbolically gaining control, and realistically reducing stress. Note that radio and television coverage in Dallas of Arthur Mitchell, an African American *danseur* and choreographer, made the history of ballet as a European tradition—formerly studied, performed, and viewed only by whites—common knowledge. News commentators repeatedly said that until Mitchell founded the Dance Theatre of Harlem, there were few black ballet dancers. Mitchell came to Dallas periodically to teach, and Pacesetter offered extracurricular ballet classes. In this way, blacks learned the ballet rules well enough not only to execute them but also to break them.

The child appeared to engage in sympathetic magic in the sense that she symbolically enacted, through body motion, wished-for behavior. When she collapsed her arabesque pose in lieu of concluding it with the traditional ballet aplomb, she seemed to symbolize or, with the compelling power of metaphor, to affect the white teacher's complete downfall from authority.

**Illustration 2**
At least once a week I saw one to six black children at a time spontaneously dance a few steps in short sequences in a variety of situations both inside and outside the classroom in ways that did not disrupt formal teaching and learning. For example, as a second-grade class was being dismissed, one black boy exited performing a Charleston step three times. This was the same step the black girl performed in the first illustration. After the first boy exited, a second black boy followed, performing the same movement phrase. The sequence occurred repeatedly until six black boys had left the classroom. In a fourth-grade music class, several black boys bebopped to the admiring looks of their peers. One black boy walked with exaggerated hip shifts, his upper and lower torso moving in opposition; another boy walked about while shimmying his shoulder blades. A third sat snapping his fingers and then got up and performed a step-kick

walking dance sequence. A fourth boy shook his arms and rippled his torso. As a sixth-grade class was going through the halls to the cafeteria, several black boys and girls performed a variety of dance movement phrases. At Pacesetter I never saw white children dancing spontaneously.

What specifically triggered the children's dance movements in the classrooms and halls was uncertain. For some children who find structured classroom activities incompatible with their capabilities or moods, dancing may be cathartic, a release of pent-up energy after adhering to a formal academic regime. In black folklore, the arts have a long history of providing solace and support. About the black community, black dancer and singer Bessie Jones recalls, "We'd dance awhile to rest ourselves."[15] Some kids were just having fun.

**Illustration 3**

During recess outdoors on a warm sunny day, groups of black girls spontaneously organized dance cheers, ring plays, and line plays that combined dance and song. Using the spatial form of children's dances probably of British origin and learned from white Americans, the children meshed the African style of loose, flexible torso, extending and flexing knees with an easy breathing quality, shuffling steps, and pelvic swings and thrusts to create syncretistic dances of the sort called ring and line plays.[16] Either the leader sang a phrase that the group answered or the leader led the performers. Movements accompanied and accented the song text or illustrated it. Hand clapping or other body percussion punctuated the performance to create a syncopated rhythm within the song and dance. In one instance, when a white girl wished to join the black girls in one of the dances, a black girl stepped back, put her hands on her hips, looked the white girl up and down about the hips and feet, and with a quizzical look and scowl said loudly for all to hear: "Show me you can dance!" Everyone watched as the white girl withdrew to the sidelines.

Later, a different white girl joined the "Check Me" ring play, in which the name of each participant in the circle was singled out in turn, going to the right. One girl's name was called by the girl standing to her immediate left; she identified herself, sang a refrain, and then called on the next girl to her right.

Check [clap], check [clap], check [clap]
My name is Tina.
I am a Pisces.
I want you to [clap]
check, check, check,
to check out Bridgette.
Check [clap], check [clap], check.
My name is Bridgette . . .

When it was the white girl's turn to be called, the black girl just passed her by and called the name of the next black girl. Rejected, the white girl called out, "I can do it, too!" No one paid attention.

In these dances, black pride, identity, boundaries, and neighborhood loyalty seemed to coalesce. By recognizing only blacks, the participants manifested in-group bonding in an arena in which they excelled, a response to the stressors of past white oppression and exclusion of African Americans. Their dancing suggests a way of coping with a future of racial separation possibly carried on as in the past—or even a reversal of power relations, in which blacks are superior to whites. The white audience is put on its mettle. Perhaps the black girls' dances are similar to the slaves' animal-trickster tales in which the weaker animal bests the stronger through its wits. The tales afforded their creators psychic relief, an arena of mastery, and a vision of a possible future.

## Afterword

From Africa to America, we have seen how dance is an autogenic medium to resist the negative effects of stress and to cope with stress in a remedial way. The dance may communicate messages of displeasure with situations that call for resolution. People of all ages express themselves through dance.

In presenting the case of the women's war, I have suggested that although Ubakala men dominate the traditional political organization and ritual of the egalitarian society, and its pattern of tracing descent through the paternal side and the tradition that the family resides among the husband's kin, Ubakala women also have power. They perpetuate the husband's lineage, integrate villages through marital ties, and mediate imbalances in social life as viewed from the perspective of Ubakala values. Rather than being a muted group, the women express their wishes and power in dance-plays, attempting to resist or reduce stress. The women can transform the dance-play performances into persuasive social protest with boycotts called "sitting on a man" and dance and sing their grievances. However, when their dance-play communication goes unheeded, the women can switch from playfully dancing to violently waging war—their ultimate means of enforcing their will. The 1929 women's war was a dramatic extension of the traditional method women used to settle grievances with men who acted badly toward them.

The Dallas case illustrates that children often do not feel comfortable participating in arenas where they sense that they are not welcome, they are unlikely to perform well, or the competition is unfairly matched. Thus the black children staked out their own turf, as ethnic minorities have always done. One consequence of the black dances is that the white children have been given the outsider status in informal children-delineated performance arenas at Pacesetter that blacks have traditionally had in broader arenas of life. By focusing on power through high-energy dances, the girls suggested role reversal in the wider society. What the national context offers in prestige for whites, the local arena offers in recognition and power for blacks.

It is fascinating that the African American schoolchildren in Dallas had no direct contact with the Ubakala performers in Nigeria, yet the stress-related pattern of protest through dance that is widespread and historically rooted in Africa appears to have survived in the new land.

# CHAPTER SEVEN

~

# Revitalizing the Past and Facing the Future

Groups often turn to their cultural roots when confronted with the stress of change and negative contact with other groups. These turnings to earlier practices usually mean that these traditions become modified in light of contemporary issues. In Kenya, the Kikuyu traditionally danced to proclaim a new government; a war dance was held in every district. Words from a drafted constitution were embodied in song and dance. Nor surprisingly, the Kikuyu danced in the capital, Nairobi, to celebrate Independence Day in 1963, the end of British colonial rule. Others groups displayed their physical fitness and dexterity in handling spears and shields that they had relied on in the past and that had brought them recognition and praise.

Religious or secular responses that incorporate dance appear to be attempts to revitalize what is perceived to have had positive benefits in the past. Sometimes new dance forms evolve in which people reduce the stress of a sense of inferiority by identifying with the aggressor, accommodating rather than submitting, or resisting through defiant nonverbal expression. These dances provide arenas of self-affirmation and self-mastery in situations in which people feel they have lost political and economic power. The dancing is usually framed, highlighted, or prepared for with religious offerings or other acts, such as using drugs, altering eating, resting, and sexual patterns, and submitting to social isolation, that distinguish the everyday from the dance performance. In this chapter I'll present illustrative cases from West and East Africa, North America, and Mexico.

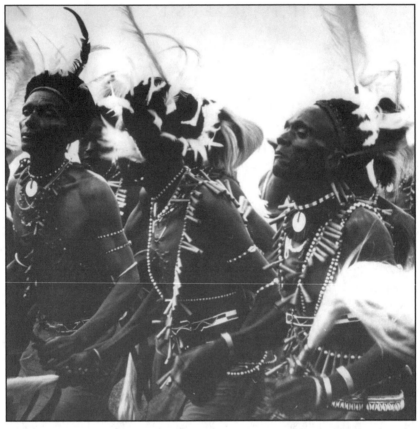

**Figure 7.1.** Dancing the 1963 Constitution (Photo of Kikuyu Celebrating Kenya's Independence by William John Hanna)

## Bwiti

In response to multiple stressors during the twentieth century, the Fang of Gabon developed Bwiti, a syncretistic cult, or revitalization movement, that draws upon both indigenous African and foreign Christian rituals and beliefs. James Fernandez's extensive study of Bwiti[1] provides the following information. The dance in Bwiti religious action and mythology stems from the Fang rather than the colonialist Christian tradition. Differing in some respects from the dances performed in other realms of Fang social life, the skillful Bwiti dance performance is believed to be essential to obtain the blessing and benevolence of the supernatural. So cult leaders paint the feet of their members with a special paste to ensure flawless dancing.

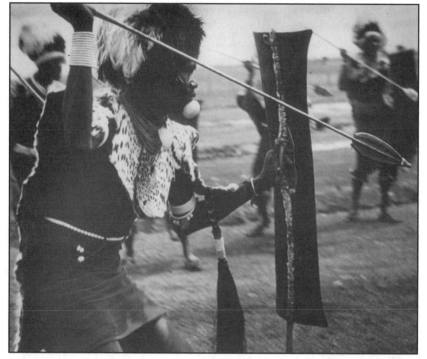

**Figure 7.2. Remembering War Preparation (Photo of Luo by William John Hanna)**

Bwiti evolved in response to the Fangs' need for protection and revitaliza-tion as a result of the pressures of French colonial domination and missionary evangelization. The Fang experienced restricted personal expression and feel-ing states, and in the 1930s, Bwiti took a clandestine form because of the French objection to some of its practices.

Catalysts for the development of Bwiti were harrowing threats of periodic famine, disease, and population decline coupled with occasional confronta-tions with colonial administrators or religious missionaries. In one Fang con-gregation, thirty out of fifty-six males had no children. And some, such as Ekang, had few offspring. His fourth and last wife produced two surviving daughters In such infertile unions, every pregnancy was carefully watched and accusations of witchcraft were often made by one wife against the other in the event of miscarriage or the death of an infant. European contact with the Fang led to an increased scale of social and spiritual relationships in which "the reality of the far away has come to challenge what was previously the overriding reality of the near and the parochial. With Christianity came the challenge to the old traditional protectively benevolent powers of the below by the missionary message of divinity in the above."[2]

The Bwiti cult placates and reconciles those who are troubled and alienated from their usual relationships with both gods and men. Bwiti "satisfies by providing a whole experience for those to whom life does not provide enough of anything they feel they need, who feel they are not taking part or who, at best, feel they are allotted an insignificant part of the whole."[3] Those well versed in Bwiti lore create for their membership a "pleasure dome" where they feel at home. Bwiti ties together what witches and sorcerers and the agents of the colonial world and simply modern times have torn asunder Under such stressful conditions, men and women bereft of the solidarity and strength of the group feel preyed upon.[4]

This telling reason for joining Bwiti may well account for why dance works, or is efficacious, for many people: "I was a Christian but I found no truth in it. Christianity is the religion of the whites. It is the whites who have brought us the Cross and the Book. All the things in their religion one hears by the ears. But we Fang do not learn that way. We learn by the eyes. To counter the sense of bodily isolation and decay and vulnerability to evil, and a burdensome sense of accumulating impurities, there is vigorous purifying engagement in ritual that is followed by ecstatic bodily transcendence.[5]

The Fang represented the healthiness of flow in the social body by extension of their understanding of the importance of flow in the personal body. One act in Bwiti moves away from the quality of "bad body" to the quality of "clean body," or "clean heartedness." Because sexual appetite and indulgence are primary causes of bad body, the ritual requires abstention and purity.

Cult leaders say that one of the purposes of the all-night dancing is to sacrifice to God and to the ancestors the sexual pleasure of the body, although at the metaphoric and symbolic level of culture activity there is plenty of sexuality being represented.[6] The all-night ceremonies end at dawn with dances that encircle the ancestors' welcoming hut and dances of compressed circles of "one heartedness" performed in front of the hut, on the edge of the forest, and down in the center of the nearby stream. In a state of deep fatigue from the night's exertion, most of the members feel a sense of purity at having rid their bodies of impurities through the vertiginous activity and copious perspiration.[7]

However, sexuality has its place in Bwiti, since one of its key purposes is the ritual inducement of fertility. The corporeal symbolism, carried out in the assimilation of the chapel itself to a body, appears in the men's entrance dances. After the women Bwiti participants enter the chapel, the men arrive at the birth entrance of the chapel and halt there. The leaders place their hands on the thatch, or the lintel piece above them. Then the entire group in close-packed formation backs up and moves forward again in successive surges. The group penetrates more deeply into the chapel until the men are entirely within and ready to begin circle dances. These actions at the birth entrance represent the difficult birth of men out of natural life into the spiritual world of the ancestors, and also the entrance of the male organ into the female body.[8]

The Bwiti dance leader has taken on the name of the old Fang diviner and witch doctor, whose task was to penetrate the unseen in favor of the afflicted. "The Bwiti *nganga*, by leading the membership fruitfully down the path of birth and death, does, in effect, like the *nganga* of old, enable them to penetrate into the unseen, to pass over into the land of the dead and, in so doing, to assuage their afflictions. Dancing successfully down the path of birth and death demands orderliness within the chapel and . . . the exclusion of agents of disorderliness such as witches and other errant supernaturals."[9]

The pounding chants, songs, and dances create a performance intensity. With various meanings at different times of the evening, the *obango* dance generally refers to the turmoil of the soul as it either enters the body, at birth, or departs it, at death. "*Obango* has the meaning, if not of sexual passion, at least of ecstatic activity with fertile consequences. The women team dancers shake their buttocks, laden with sleigh bells, which represent the child in the womb, "while their shaking of their buttocks is directly enticing."[10]

Staying up the whole night is tiring; vigorous dancing, too, further exhausts Bwiti members. They take *eboga*, a crop common to the equatorial forest that has psychotropic properties. It produces a euphoric insomnia and energy. "Members often say that the *eboga* taken in this way also lightens their bodies so that they can float through their ritual dances."[11]

Thus the ancestral Bwiti cult is a response to stress, an effort to reduce and escape stress, if only temporarily. In its ritual practices, especially the prominently featured dancing, Bwiti symbolically enacts wished-for resolution of personal and social difficulties. There is also the reality of people coming together as a support group and physically expelling accumulated tensions—energy mobilized by the stress response and not otherwise released—through the all-night dancing in a state of altered sensibility that results from the excitement, fatigue, and drugs.

## American Ghost Dance

Native Americans have experienced years of stress from white political and economic domination. Defeat, the recognized inability to counteract the invaders and the ensuing poverty, seemed to fortify the American Indians' faith

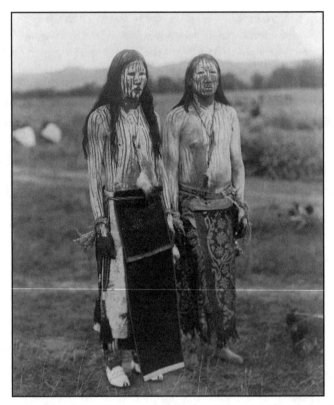

**Figure 7.3.  Identity (Photo of Cheyenne Sun Dance Pledgers by Edward S. Curtis, 1920, Courtesy of Library of Congress, Prints and Photographs Division)**

to practice ritual designed to hasten world renewal. The American Indians have historically looked to the supernatural to accomplish what they could not do by themselves. Dance, such as in the Ghost Dance religion, is part of a repeated florescence of American Indian religious revivals that reaffirm traditional values and enlist ancient religious beliefs in periodic renewal of the world as a means of attempting to effect change.

The Northern Paiute and peoples of the Northwest Plateau believed that ceremonies involving group dancing, a visible index of ethnic and political alliances and actions, had power to end the deprivation that resulted from their defeat at the hands of whites and bring about a return to the earlier days of American Indian prosperity, specifically the restoration of lost lands.

By the 1880s, the United States government had managed to confine almost all the Indians on reservations on poor land, renege on providing adequate rations and supplies that had been guaranteed them by the treaties, and support an Indian Bureau that was rampant with graft and corruption. In response to such deprivation, a Paiute Indian named Wovoka announced in 1889 that he was the messiah, come to earth to prepare the Indians for their salvation through the Ghost Dance. In order to attract acculturated American Indians who had converted to Christianity, the Ghost Dance religion of the late nineteenth century incorporated Christian teachings of the millennium and the second coming of Christ. Modern transportation and communication spread the ideas.[12]

The dance commonly commenced in the afternoon or after sundown. It took the Indians about two hours to paint and dress themselves. Then the leaders walked to the dance place and joined hands to form a small circle and begin to sing. As their song reach full voice, people came singly and in groups from the several tipis to join the circle until as many as fifty to five hundred men, women, and children were dancing. Unlike other Indian dances with fast steps and loud drumming, the Ghost Dance consisted of slow shuffling movements following the course of the sun. It would be performed for four or five days and was accompanied by singing and chanting, occasions, when, dance may have acted as a demographic revitalization movement.[13] The Ghost Dance occurred at the time of a low in the American Indian population. Through disease, relocation, starvation, genocide, and social and cultural destruction, the American Indian population was decimated to an 1890 nadir of a mere 228,000 from a total of about 600,000 in 1800. Virtually all smaller tribes participated in the dance, which was believed to return deceased American Indian people to life. A primary objective of the Ghost Dance was the resurrection of the American Indians' ancestors by returning the spirits of the dead from the spirit world to the terrestrial world.[14]

The unity and fervor that the Ghost Dance inspired, however, spurred only fear and hysteria among white settlers. This ultimately contributed to the events in 1890, which culminated in the massacre at Wounded Knee and the demise of the Ghost Dance.

## Coast Salish Spirit Dancing

Aboriginal-style winter Spirit Dancing resurged in the 1970s among the Nooksack of western Washington and more generally among other surrounding Coast Salish groups. Spirit Dancing had been declining since the advent of Christianity. The initial contact between American Indians and Europeans had resulted in positive, rewarding exchange relationships. Christianity made inroads, and intermarriage occurred. But agricultural exploitation was incompatible with American Indian traditions of hunting, fishing, and gathering, and the onslaught of European-carried diseases hurt the American Indians, whose immune systems offered little resistance. Then European attitudes turned against the American Indians, whom they viewed as obstacles to progress. As a result, the American Indians' aggressive adaptation evolved into passive nonparticipation in the white economy, and their consequent poverty. The increased participation in the traditional ceremonial rituals gave people an opportunity to affirm their worth as individuals and as American Indians in a situation in which they have progressively lost economic autonomy and have had to depend on the white welfare system.[15] The revival of the seasonal ceremonial Spirit Dancing is part of the trend toward celebrating ethnic traditions and joining cult-like religious movements in response to stress. Spirit Dancing persists among American Indians because it expresses and reconciles major cultural values and is pleasurable, offering the opportunity for spontaneity and emotional release through a trance experience.

Prior to their contact with whites, the American Indians exchanged food surpluses for wealth items through potlatch ceremonies. The Nooksack worldview held that humanity was set apart from nature. In order to exploit the natural environment of salmon, saltwater fish, land animals, and edible roots and berries, a person needed to communicate with the supernatural realm. The vehicle for supernatural contact was a person's own vision, in which the spirit endowed the person with a song and dance as visible proof of this contact and the means to mobilize the spirit's power. This communication was considered dangerous, and contact could be achieved only if the supplicant purged her- or himself of the taint of human existence by bathing, fasting, taking emetics, and submitting to social isolation. Public performance of the dance showed the strength of a person's power and thus marked the individual's role and status.

In contemporary Nooksack religious belief, the key spiritual entity is the soul, an ever-present danger to its owner and others. Because the soul is light and easily dislodged from its owner, loss of the soul is believed to cause illness to the owner as well as the person who has inadvertently attracted it.[16] A sudden fright or great sorrow will cause the soul to fly away, or it can be stolen intentionally or unintentionally. Moreover ghosts or persons with strong spirit power can steal the soul, or a person with a strong spirit power may unwittingly attract a soul after it has been dislodged from its owner. Consequently, children should be kept away from places where powerful spirit forces are present. Children are not allowed on the floor of a dance house during a winter dance or permitted to get close to a new dancer.

Old patterns have changed. Instead of questing for power in adolescence and waiting five or ten years before dancing publicly, postadolescent teenagers and older people now can become dance participants. Today, instead of receiving a unique vision, most participants now receive a vision that previously had been in the family. The tutelary of a deceased relative selects an appropriate candidate and troubles the individual until the person accepts the vision and manifests contact with this spirit through the dance. A spontaneous vision may come through sickness, sorrow, dreaming, or through dancers who grab individuals and infuse them with power.

Initiation into the dance creates a new social role for the candidate and mediates the contradiction between the principles of rugged individualism and of mutual support, cooperation, and interdependence of kin. Initiation begins with a rite of separation that lasts from four to ten days, during which the new dancer is purified and helped with his or her song. The following transition or liminal period lasts the rest of the dance season.

Dancing is necessary to avoid supernatural and social penalties. Often the words of the song and movements of the dance are stylized mimicry of the tutelary. The American Indians believe illnesses respond to spirit dancing; magic spells may be used by dancers as protection in initiation and from hostile shamans.

Participants in the contemporary winter ceremonials belong to some local group, which in turn belongs to the larger dance community. Seating in the dance house is organized according to village or reservation unit, as is the order of performance. The dance thus perpetuates intervillage ties, intensifies the bonds of the local unit, and promotes social solidarity and identity. A person needs her or his spouse's help to dance the spirit power properly. Thus the dance reinforces marital ties and the idea of family closeness as buffers to stressors.

The Nooksack require correct decorum in the dance. A dancer who falls, a drummer who errs and confuses a dancer, or a dancer who loses part of the dance costume, suggest ritual injury. Then the performer and his or her kin and their local group all lose face.

There are three kinds of invasions by an alien spiritual entity: a hostile spirit, friendly spirit, or strange soul who causes illnesses. Many dancers begin possession by crying or sighing in distress; the onset may cause a chest pain, which dissipates when they dance. Entranced dancers perform a specific song and dance. The Coast Salish view the Spirit Dancer's trance as a special case of the panhuman capacity to seek altered states of consciousness.

Salish dancing allows catharsis, the release of pent-up emotional tensions, in a culturally valued and socially approved way that gives the performer a sense of mastery and autonomy. Self-confidence generated by the knowledge that one is able to tap genuine supernatural resources offers the individual valid evidence of being special as an American Indian in a world exclusive to the American Indians.

# The Gourd Dance

Formerly performed exclusively by the Comanche, Wind River Shoshone, Cheyenne, Arapaho, Omaha, and other warrior societies, the Gourd Dance has become popular also with groups whose ancestors never performed it. The Kiowa and Comanche group dance societies' invitational performances in the 1960s at the Tulsa, Okalahoma, powwow and other large intertribal urban powwows led to a momentous spread of the dance throughout the state of Oklahoma among twenty additional Native American groups and even beyond Arizona and New Mexico.

The dance provides a vehicle by which Native Americans can express their identity.[17] A Kiowa informant says about the dance, "It's just like prayer songs, it just makes you happy, and makes people feel good.... We want to help the people who may be in mourning and want to come back, or may be sick, or have troubles."[18] Clearly the Gourd Dance is believed to have healing qualities.

Singers sit in the center of the dance arena; male dancers sit on benches around the periphery. One bench is reserved for the female head dancer and her assistants. The other female dancers and spectators sit in folding chairs behind the benches. An invocation precedes the dance, which begins gradually with songs accompanied by dancers shaking their gourds softly in time with the music. The head male dancer and some of his friends rise and dance in place, still shaking their gourds softly. They flex their knees on the loud beat and straighten them, sometimes with a slight bumping of the heels, on the soft beat. At times the dancers bend slightly forward from the waist while swooping an arm toward the floor. Other dancers gradually rise and join the performers as the beat picks up considerably. At the end of a song, signaled by a flurry of fast drumbeats, all of the dancers raise their gourds high into the air and vibrate them. The tempo and excitement build up an electric atmosphere.

## Danza de la Conquista

Originating in the Mexican states of Queretaro and Guanajuato in response to the Spanish conquest in the sixteenth century, dance groups known as *concheros, danza Chicimeca, danza Azteca,* and *danza de la conquista* continue to exist. The groups, also called crisis cults, are syncretistic attempts to create pride in their cultural identity and new forms of social integration in a changing milieu. Part of handling the stress of conquest and its lingering aftermath is identification with the aggressor.[19] Mostly from the laborer and shoeshine occupations, the dancers are at the low end of the socioeconomic scale. They adopt the nomenclature of the Spanish military hierarchy and perform dances reenacting the conquest. The dances were derived from the Spanish representations of Moors and Christians. Women, the elderly, and children, as well as men, perform the warlike dances.[20]

## Beni Ngoma

Popular in East Africa (urban and rural Kenya, Tanzania, Zambia, and Rhodesia, now called Zimbabwe), Beni was, from at least 1890 to 1970, a popular versatile team dance (*ngoma*) with essentially urban origins. The dance has recognizable features of modernity (European dress, military band, drill, organization, and a hierarchy of officers with European titles), besides traditional African competitiveness.[21] The dance is enmeshed in the stresses related to more than one hundred years of history, including colonial occupation, display of European military power, the devastation of World War I, the great depression and protest, the development of strike action, and the impact of World War II.

Beni, with elements of resistance, compulsion, and protest, is a medium of balancing emasculation and creativity, accommodation and independence. It is "one of a series of brass-band responses by people in a transitional period from pre-industrial to industrial society," comparable to the brass-band competitions of the Lancashire industrial village in England, band processions of eighteenth-century Jamaica, or bands of Brazil.[22]

An indigenous form that selectively borrows from the powerful, Beni is an accommodation rather than a submission. This dance allows a display of self-respect and self-confidence in communal values based on locality, ethnicity, tribal divisions, or class against others in a continuing tradition of communal dance competitions. These groups have elaborate ranks, displays of military skills, opportunities for innovation, achievement of high rank, and the exercise of patronage for high status.

## Afterword

I have sketched some dances of peoples who have felt stressed by the impact of domination by a more-powerful group through colonization or defeat in war. When suffering a loss of economic and social power and self-esteem, besides the stressors of natural disasters and life in general, people often find succor through the dance medium. Bwiti and Beni Ngoma dances from Africa and the Ghost Dance, Coast Salish Spirit Dancing, Gourd Dance, and *danza de la conquista* from the Americas are examples of means these groups chose to resist, reduce, or escape stress. The dances provided an outlet for energy mobilized in the stress response. Cathartic with avenues of altered states of consciousness, including trance, the dances offer opportunities to confront the stressors through physical and cognitive structuring in which the outcomes are favorable. Individuals find strength in the self-mastery required in dance and receive the support of others in cohesive group dancing, which provides a kind of therapy. The effort to revitalize what was perceived in the past to have had positive benefit blends with elements of the new. Dance always changes. Identifying with the aggressor, accommodating rather than submitting, or resisting through defiant nonverbal dance expression offers arenas of self and group affirmation.

# PART III

# WESTERN DANCE-STRESS RELATIONS

The palette of human experience in dance-stress connections is multicolored throughout history and across cultures. What are dance themes and practices in contemporary Western society that help people resist, reduce, and escape stress or, indeed, induce stress? Dance images in social, educational, work, therapeutic, and theater settings that are broadcast over television, cable, and the Internet reach nearly the entire United States and much of the world can have a significant impact. Before the advent of these broadcast possibilities, theater dance was the province of a narrow population of performers and ticket-paying theater goers, and aerobic dance was taught in patron-paying gyms and recreational centers. Dancers create moving narratives or poetic images that allow both dancer and observer to confront and work through stressful situations. The images may be a commentary or critique. Performers pay tribute to human fortitude as they express the sense of doing something and being in control, even if changing a situation is unlikely. Of course, dance is entertainment that permits diversion and escape from stressors.

In professional and amateur settings, dance can release energy mobilized by the fight-flight stress response that is otherwise restrained. Pursuing a dance career has great rewards, but as with many occupations, there are stressors, many of which are unique to the pursuit of dance as a livelihood. Amateur dancing has fewer hazards because it is a more relaxed endeavor.

Dance is more than a theater art and a form of leisure. It is also an explicit form of healing that is often part of mainstream medical treatment programs.

~

## CHAPTER EIGHT

# "Playing" Onstage in Western Theatrical Dance

Modern Western society has an advanced technology and a generally high quality of life that contrast with the situations of past societies, some Western minorities, and many non-Western countries today. Yet, as members of the same species, people in contemporary society are affected by similar stressors related to life-cycle vicissitudes and social exchanges. We all need love and hope for acceptance. A prevalent leitmotif in the human record is that through dance, themes such as poverty, death, sexuality, gender roles, violation of societal norms, drug abuse, discrimination, and oppression, performers and observers attempt to cope with anxieties and fears. Stories from the Bible and the Hindu epics are enacted in dance. Fairy tales, too.

Kinetic discourse allows you to examine past, present, or anticipated events to deflect, palliate, or flee stress. The staged performance of wordless poems or narratives about stressors is pretend, play, and therefore distant and less threatening than the real world. When you scrutinize dance images that illuminate the human outlook, the revelations about self or society may be like those that occur in psychotherapy, including dance therapy. You may gain insight that moves you to evaluate problems, consider resolutions, and act in a constructive way outside the dance setting. Indeed, it is the potency of emotional engagement in the dance that leads many totalitarian countries to attempt to control dance and other arts, because they fear the arts will arouse unrestrained passions. Uninhibited ecstasy, or its symbolic representations, can remind the constrained of how restricted they are. A political critique against a stress-inducing regime can be produced in dance texts not so much by an inherent or explicit political opposition as by a symbolic subversion

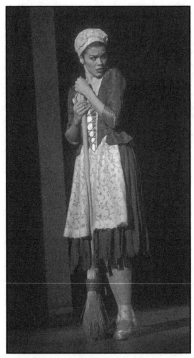

**Figure 8.1.** *Cinderella* **(Photo of Michelle Jimenez, Washington Ballet, by Carol Pratt)**

within the art form. The presentation of tragedy also sends a message of "be cool, this is life, get on with it." The live dancer embodying these concepts does not succumb but manifests resistance to the stress of tragedy. The ballet *Cinderella* portrays poverty, discrimination, meanness, but also escape through dance. Downtrodden, Cinderella meets her savior Prince Charming at a ball.

Yin Mei's *Nomad: The River* tells of her childhood clouded by China's Cultural Revolution, but blessed by dreams of a world beyond.

Of course, much theater dance is entertainment and enchantment, or play with form in and of itself—a diversion and escape from stress. Thus for many dance participants, dance is devoid of serious meaning. Yet in serious dances, there can be humorous interludes.

Some of the illustrative dances in this chapter depict overlapping themes and convey multiple meanings. Dancers and dance viewers have their own take on a performance based on personal imagination, experience, and knowledge. Moreover, the same work performed by different dancers may send different messages.

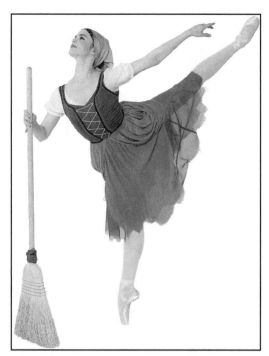

Figure 8.2. *Cinderella* (Photo of Michelle Jimenez, Washington Ballet, by Tony Powell)

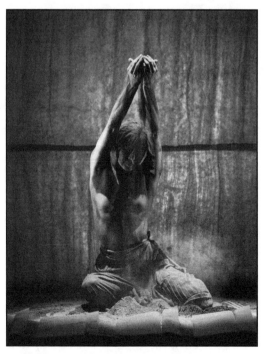

Figure 8.3. *Nomad* (Photo of Yin Mei by Charles Martin)

# Death

After the tragic death of her two children, pioneer modern dancer Isadora Duncan choreographed *Mother*, a poignant dirge for every mother who has lost a child. Martha Graham's *Death and Entrances* was inspired by the lives of the three Brontë sisters and was also about Graham and her two sisters. Jerome Robbins dedicated *Quiet City* to Joseph Duell, a principal dancer for the New York City Ballet who committed suicide. The ballet ends with groups of dancers kneeling or standing in shadows.

Robbins's *In Memory of . . .* reveals young loving couples dancing together and then experiencing unrest and inevitability. A young man who proves to be Death appears to claim one of the women, who struggles until he subdues her. George Balanchine's *Adagio Lamentoso* begins with three grieving women who dance barefoot and with loose hair. The mourners are joined by an ensemble to share with them reflections on the transitory nature of life. *Dark Elegies*, choreographed by Antony Tudor, suggests a communal ritual: through mourning, people cope with loss and death as a fact of life.

*The Duel*, choreographed by William Dollar, tells the tragedy of Tancred, the Christian warrior, and Clorinda, a pagan girl, who meet and fall in love and

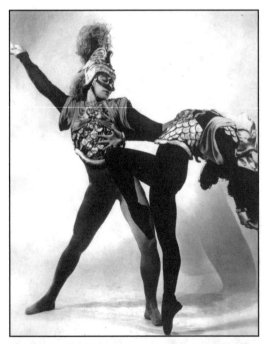

**Figure 8.4.** *The Duel* **(Francisco Moncion and Melissa Hayden, New York City Ballet. Courtesy of National Archives)**

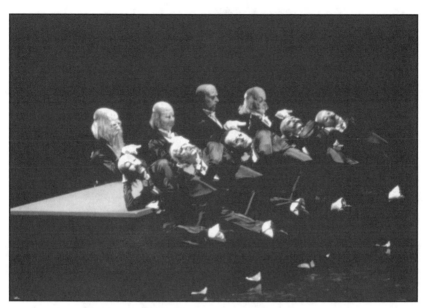

**Figure 8.5.** *Green Table* **(Photo of Joffrey Ballet by Herbert Migdoll)**

as unwitting opponents battle to the death. Eliot Feld's ballet *A Soldier's Tale* recounts a story about the horrors of war, including the pimp and prostitute who prey upon its men.

Kurt Jooss's 1932 antiwar ballet, *Green Table*, continues to be performed. Moving people to action against violence was Jooss's goal. The work delivers an overt message about duplicity, its path to war, and death. Masked diplomats suggest culpability in violence; a martial figure personifying war leads the dance of death.

In *Triumph of Death*, Flemming Flindt's choreography of nude dancers performing to a rock score dramatizes the manner in which human existence is threatened by environmental pollution, political tyranny, corruption, and cities contaminated by nuclear fallout. Nudity shows the common currency of humanity.

Alvin Ailey's *Flowers* reflects on the doomed black-influenced blues-rock singer Janis Joplin, who became a drug addict and died of an overdose. *Undertow*, by Tudor, tells a story of a boy driven to murder. Crammed with nervous movement or urban restlessness and tension, the ballet presents scenes of brutal sex, hypocrisy, and other evils.

The epic plight of the American Indian, including the slaughter and degrading violence against Indian women, is the theme of Michael Smuin's *A Song of a Dead Warrior*. It has a cast of thirty-one dancers and spectacular

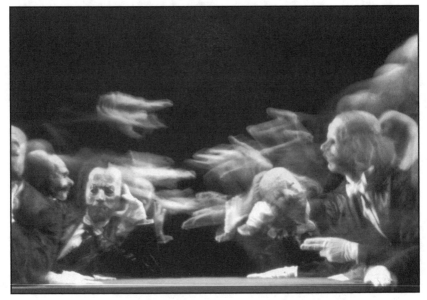

**Figure 8.6.** *Green Table* **(Photo of Joffrey Ballet by Herbert Migdoll)**

effects—ghostlike sheriffs standing twenty feet tall and huge photographic blow-ups of bison. Smuin was inspired by the two-year occupation of the Alcatraz penitentiary by a group of American Indian dissidents and their leader, a youth named Richard Oakes. He is portrayed as a young brave who dreams of ancestral rites and glory. While attending a reservation dance, he and his sweetheart are attacked by state troopers, who rape and murder the girl. Overwhelmed, he becomes an alcoholic. We see the young man savagely beaten by pool-hall thugs. Another ancestral vision comes to him. Inspired by his chiefly forebears, he rouses himself to fight, kill, and scalp the sheriff in an act born of revenge. His efforts are, however, to no avail; the troopers shoot him down.

## Survivors

José Limon's *Missa Brevis* presents a chorus of dancers mourning in a bombed-out church. Gerald Arpino's *The Clowns* is a parable about human survival in the face of nuclear war and its aftermath. The ballet explores cycles of rebirth and destruction, adding a comic twist to the nightmarish theme: circus figures comment upon the ultimate ludicrousness of nuclear Armageddon. Technologically innovative in using huge clear plastic balloons and pillows, Arpino shows technology gone awry as it envelopes the clowns.

Butoh, the "dance of darkness," originated in Japan and reflects the cataclysmic aftermath of the atomic bomb on Hiroshima and Nagasaki at the end of World War II. The genre, which also has roots in German expressionism, is mysterious and shocking in its portrayal of aggression, suffering, forbidden sexual passions, and human frailty. Fascinated with the grotesque and absurd, butoh founder Tatsumi Hijikata described butoh as "a mirror which thaws fear," "a corpse standing straight up in a desperate bid for life."[1] He refers to the need to annihilate memory (see chapter 1 for the discussion of VAM and SAM memory, and altering the way we think to improve mental health). Onstage, dancers appear distorted, nude, emaciated, without hair on their heads, and with a white pastelike substance covering their faces and bodies to erase humanity.[2]

Three years prior to 9/11, New York choreographer Tamar Rogoff was working on a piece about post-traumatic stress disorder, a psychological response to the horrors of war. (See prelude.) She wanted to understand her father, a veteran of World War II who experienced insomnia and claustrophobia, was

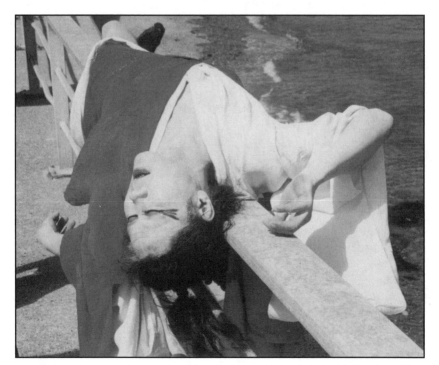

**Figure 8.7.** *Sun Circular* (Photo of butoh dancer Tadashi Endo by Connie Müller-Gödecke)

aloof, and never talked about the war or told her that he loved her. Rogoff
had discovered a box of her deceased father's letters that described his horrific experience in Burma. She and the five members of her dance company,
Tamar Rogoff Performance Projects, spent hours over a period of about nine
months at the Veterans Affairs Medical Center in Manhattan listening to five
veterans speak about their combat experiences. She learned that emotional
detachment was part of post-traumatic stress disorder. "My idea was to make
war visible, because I felt it was invisible. I was aiming toward our numbness—
like wearing camouflage clothes without thinking about what that means."[3]
After the 9/11 Pentagon and World Trade Center attacks, she realized the
veterans were talking about how to survive. Inspired by the veterans' stories,
each dancer performed a solo to the recorded voice of a veteran whose pho-
tograph appeared in the background. John McCarthy, a seventy-six-year-old
veteran of World War II, described surviving a plane crash. "In the fall of 1943,
flying still had a mystique about it, and it was glamorous. Then the day came
when we had the crash landing. We were up maybe several hundred feet with
a full high-octane gas load, and that changed my feelings a lot. I was scared to
death, and I cried out to God for help. It was horrendously frightening. I can't
describe the terror. It's just absolutely awful." The process of the dance making
was cathartic for the veterans, and they felt gratified that people cared about
the sacrifices they made for their country. The dancers, too, benefited. Hearing
the stories of a veteran who was held over a cliff by the SS, went blind, and
survived two plane crashes helped them put their own problems in perspective.

The 9/11 attacks evoked a choreographic tribute, mourning, outlet for
anger, and questioning in Vladimir Angelov's *Deep Surface*. The piece was performed live and then on film. Expressive contemporary-movement vocabulary
interweaves with documentary film footage of 9/11 to convey a kind of immedi-
acy. The choreography, includes two dancers who each raise an arm, reaching
toward the fallen towers; the group cradles a woman who leaves their embrace,
their arms left cradling nothing, symbolizing a loved one lost. Dancers look
upward and surge forward in a line formation and then retreat. In a tightly
knit group, dancers' torsos bend forward and back as if in mourning. Splayed
hands, tense bodies, vibratory movement, and burning gazes express anger.

Modern dancer Nejla Y. Yatkin was interested in people's emotional state
after 9/11. "I was seeing so much, hearing so much. I was so overwhelmed that
it felt like I was in a dream state, seeing picture after picture go by, over and
over again. During my East European tour in 2002, I interviewed artists, I came
across: what would they say to someone in their last five minutes of life? I put
the interviews in a collage. I observed people's reactions and reflections. My
piece *After* is a journey of peoples' emotional stages when they are confronted
with the thought of loss."[4]

## Repressed Sexuality and Unrequited Love

As sexual beings who seek intimate relationships, people may be stressed by less-than-ideal outcomes. Tudor's *Pillar of Fire* is a tale of repressed sexuality. Hagar, on the verge of spinsterhood, loves a man who is attracted to her younger sister. The tale of pathos eventually turns to Hagar's fulfillment. Robert Joffrey's *Remembrances* conveys the reverie of a composer's lost love through the mood of movement and music. The dance portrays romance, delight, sorrow, despair, and hope.

In *Jardin aux Lilas* Tudor reveals the pain of charming, gracious, and affluent people bound by restrictive social conventions. The misalliance of external material prosperity and social appearances is juxtaposed to interpersonal feelings and misery. The heroine, Caroline, must forsake her true love, who is not of her social class, and enter into a marriage of convenience. Playing out secrets of stealthy approaches and sad partings, the ballet could be viewed metaphorically as a comment against any arbitrary constraints.

## Americana, Sin, Perversity, and Alienation

With a merciless eye for Americana, choreographer Paul Taylor confronts acts of duplicity and sexual perversity, from spousal abuse and wife swapping to incest. In Taylor's mordant critiques, society's taboos surface, as do the stresses of violating them. *American Genesis* is an evening-length biblical-historical-allegorical dance with period dance styles used to evoke behavior of each era. The hillbilly Eden, the bouncy cakewalk, and minstrel dancing in the "Flood" section convey something of the innocence of Adam and Eve in the garden and the spirited irresponsibility of Noah's children. In the "Before Eden" section, an air of seductiveness and sexual intrigue permeates the contained manners of a minuet. Taylor reveals his liberated views of sex as women play male roles or appear as angels with male names, Adam and Eve engage in a ménage à trois, and some early Americans are caught wife swapping. A character may show disapproval while another touts the benefits of sin. The "West of Eden" section tells the story of an orgy of lust, rape, and fratricide. Cain and Abel receive impartial comfort at the end by one elder; two other elders who instigate the situation wash their hands of all responsibility.[5]

Taylor's *Big Bertha* is simultaneously humorous, macabre, garish, and provocative. An all-American middle-class family visiting a fair in 1946 becomes mesmerized into bestiality by Bertha, a huge, gaudy mechanical carnival doll of a nickelodeon. It incessantly plays sentimental waltzes and marches. The family begins to dance shyly and politely for each other. Suddenly the father becomes agitated and slaps his wife. Then the whole family turns into fiends. The father starts fondling his daughter and then drags her off to the bushes. At first she is shocked but soon appears to want another such episode. The mother meanwhile has become a hussy and, like a stripper, taken off her outer clothes, and in her red fringed underwear she stands on a chair, wiggling.[6]

William Forsythe's ballet *Say Bye-Bye*, without literally depicting physical abuse, is aggressive, powerful and downright hysterical, both a pop ballet and a sharp commentary on Western contemporary society. The entire atmosphere, with loud sound, high-energy flinging movement and stylized lack of emotion among the characters, "sports an alienation motif," condemning "the mindless joyless gaiety it depicts." Onstage,

> six men, in white shirts and ties (but threatening in their tic of punching one black-leather-gloved hand into another) and six women in black, bounce, dance and neck as if there were no tomorrow . . . a seventh woman, neurotic in her more conservative black dress . . . attempts to drown out the din. She screams "Stop," twitches and retreats to the symbol of [an] American car . . . parked in a corner of . . . [the] three-walled no-exit set. . . . The controlling image, actual and metaphoric, is of going nowhere. Abruptly, the ballet comes to an end.[7]

When the sexual revolution occurred in the 1960s, it expanded the range of partners with whom one could have intimate relations. Sexual intercourse not only increased but became detached and impersonal, creating stress for some people. Choreographer Robert Joffrey's intense, sexual, and psychedelic ballet *Astarte* captures this ethos. From his seat in the audience, a male dancer reaches the stage, where he peels to his shorts and then engages in simulated lovemaking with his partner—while on a huge, billowing high screen above, a film gives an interpretive duplication of their actions onstage. The filmed images of the dancers are dematerialized, larger and more variable than life. In the duet, each partner seems to be responding to his or her own needs rather than to the preferences of the other or even a sense of the other's space. Remote and unyielding, she interacts with him in his desire. "Each one, separately, reaches a climax that is expressed in destructive fury. Each one, in a sense, rapes the other. When they move apart at the end, neither one has been satisfied or changed," writes critic Marcia Siegel.[8]

Anna Sokolow, a believer in the rebelliousness of modern dance, argues that dances should draw upon the stress of reality to provoke and shock. Her dance *Rooms* is about the loneliness of and lack of communication between people in a big city. Chairs substitute for rooms, each dancer on one, isolated from all the others, though physically close to them.

Eugene Loring's choreography for *Billy the Kid* is based on American folk tales from the Wild West. The ballet captures the era of westward expansion

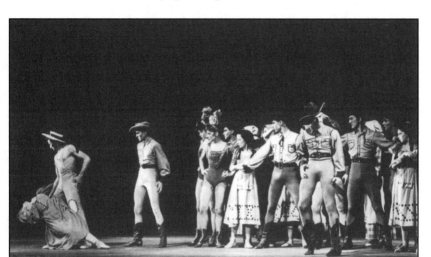

**Figure 8.8.** *Billy the kid.* **(Photo courtesy of National Archives)**

with cowboys riding imaginary horses, pioneer women, Mexicans, saloon girls, card games, and roaring gunfights. According to one story, Billy is the legendary William H. Bonney, who killed a man for every year of his life. Other tales portray Billy as a courageous, generous, engaging boy. As heroes of western movies would spin their revolvers on a finger prior to pulling the trigger, Billy's pirouettes are an expression of bravado. He is ultimately shot by the sheriff.

"The golden years" is a bogus euphemism for the agonies of growing old in America. Although choreographers rarely concern themselves with this stressful problem, D. J. McDonald's *Nocturnes* depicts a middle-aged couple trying to recapture the romance of youth with bittersweet success. His *Grandfather Songs* includes different dancers taking turns portraying an elderly man whose life consists of listening to the radio in reverie.

## Oppression of Blacks

Because of segregation, during the 20th century, blacks had their own theater circuits. When desegregation occurred, blacks began to present their choreography on stages along with whites. For example, Talley Beatty's *The Road of the Phoebe Snow* is evocative of the stress of life, youth, and death in the ghetto. Donald McKayle's *Rainbow 'Round My Shoulder* is an angry dance of protest against the Southern chain-gang system. The men dream of freedom and women waiting on the outside.

*Morning without Sunrise* is Eleo Pomare's danced narrative about the people of South Africa. Antiapartheid leader Nelson Mandela's statement during his imprisonment that "if things are not coming together, they are coming apart" inspired the choreography. The dance portrays the natural setting, unrest, and revolution in the black township of Soweto as well as dying revolutionaries, and the poignant contribution of women fighters.[9]

Among his various identities, especially being an artist, modern dancer Bill T. Jones uses the language of dance to reflect on being black, HIV positive, and vulnerable in an America faced with racism, homophobia, and puritanism. In his widely acclaimed *Last Supper at Uncle Tom's Cabin/The Promised Land*, first performed in 1990, Jones addressed the existential meaning of devastation. The dance celebrates the resourcefulness and courage that are necessary to perform the act of living. Jones had nearly fifty members of his company and the community onstage in the buff to show the common humanity of all people—all devoid of disguise, and unashamed, pulling together against the disparate strains of conflict.

Jones makes and performs dances about what matters to him, and he has also made the decision not to dance in order to make a statement. In support

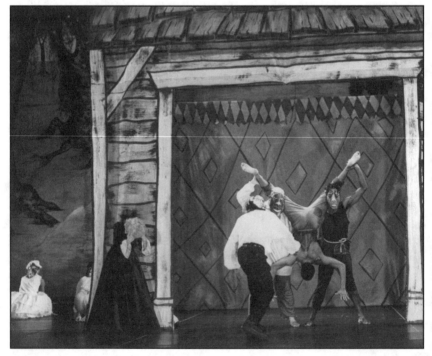

**Figure 8.9.** *Last Supper at Uncle Tom's Cabin/The Promised Land* (Photo by Martha Swope)

of an NAACP boycott, he was the first major artist to refuse to perform at the Spoleto Festival in Charleston, South Carolina, if the Confederate battle flag (symbol of racism and slavery for many people) was still flying atop the state capitol. Yet Jones also has a broad perspective in his choreography. He says his work provocatively titled *Reading, Mercy and the Artificial Nigger* "ultimately isn't about race, but about the dynamic between two people.... And if it takes a shocking title ... or my accepting a very casual use of a very hurtful word to get at something about human nature, then I have no qualms about embracing it."[10]

About his *Footprints Dressed in Red*, choreographed for Dance Theatre of Harlem, Garth Fagan says, "I wanted to say something about dancers as a community of workers and achievers, in the face of enormous pain. There's no pain in the world like the pain dancers, going at it hour after hour, day after day, and then going home perhaps to a four or five-floor walk-up—it's excruciating.... The red ... is meant to refer to the pain and blood that's a given in black culture all throughout the world."[11]

Jawole Willa Jo Zollar's Urban Bush Women modern-dance company re-sponded to the heightened political atmosphere in New York during the Re-publican convention of 2004. Recollections of civil-rights advocates inspired the hour-long piece, *Are We Democracy?* described as a "powerful segment addressed voter disenfranchisement around the nation, both organized and self-inflicted. 'Why bother?' the performers called out, along with chants of 'This is what we let happen' and 'Not my mistake, not my fault.' 'Silence'—not voting—is a form of protest!."[12]

## Women's Liberation

Establishing one's sexual and gender identities is often stressful, especially when society is in a state of flux and traditional patterns are assaulted.[13] In theater-arts dance, women have traditionally been portrayed as either vir-gin or whore; images in ballet convey male dominance through the tradi-tional *pas de deux*, in which the males support and manipulate women to allow them a greater range of movement. Female choreographers, and some male choreographers, too, have challenged the typical male-supremacist-and-female-submissive scripts that have been stressors. When artists present alter-native scenarios, not only do they release energy mobilized by the fight-flight stress response, but they also offer alternative models of behavior that suggest eliminating the stress.

Through her dances, Isadora Duncan creates an image of the female as a noble-spirited woman free to use her imagination and body as she wishes.

Senta Driver's and Bill T. Jones's choreographies reverse dancers' traditional gender roles. Men lift and flip women, and vice versa. In the dances of some female choreographers, heroic women take fate into their own hands, if only with an axe, like Lizzie Borden, who murdered her parents in order to free herself from their rules and strictures, in Agnes de Mille's *Fall River Legend*.

Martha Graham featured the settler women of America's pioneer history as protagonists in *Frontier* and *Appalachian Spring*. *Letter to the World* deals with the inner life of the New England poet Emily Dickinson and is held together by threads of her lyrical verses about her searing experiences of death and unrequited love. Graham splits the poet into two images: one who dances and one who speaks. In the corpus of her choreography, Graham deals with dominance, unbridled female passion versus duty, attraction and repulsion, and submerged guilt and open eroticism. She translates myth into an exploration of the conflict of the modern psyche. She makes classical female characters in stories such as *Oedipus Rex* human protagonists, where previously they had been the pawns of gods and men.

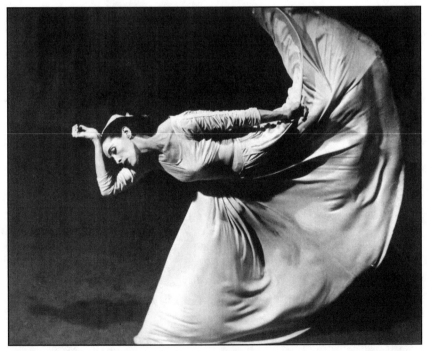

**Figure 8.10.  *Letter to the World* (Photo of Martha Graham by Barbara Morgan. Courtesy of National Archives)**

In *Clytemnestra*, as the murdered queen, Graham remembers experiences she witnessed. An angry and wild adulteress and murderer with an instinct for revenge, she at first refuses to acknowledge the evil of her misdeeds but eventually resolves personal conflict and achieves peace through self-acceptance and self-forgiveness.

Women have traditionally been a sexual object that belonged to somebody. Dance has offered voyeuristic and erotic pleasure. Whereas feminists of Isadora Duncan's generation longed for sexual freedom and viewed puritanical repression as an obstacle to their emancipation, some feminists of the 1960s and 1970s feared the sexual revolution had not liberated women so much as made them more sexually available. Postmodern choreographer Yvonne Rainer's *Trio A* illustrates the removal of the performer's seductive involvement with an audience. The performers never confront the audience, and they avert their gaze.

The 1980s heralded the advent of gentlemen's clubs, upscale strip (also called exotic, erotic, nude, and topless dance) clubs that spread nationwide and became a lightning rod for cultural conflict in America. There is a popular myth that the clubs cause crime, disease, and property depreciation. However, there is no scientific evidence for the myth.[14] The Christian right feel that such establishments challenge patriarchy and modesty (a woman belongs at home, and only a husband should see her nude body), and some feminists claim that being an object of the male gaze reinforces oppression of women. Yet, most adult-entertainment exotic dancers feel empowered. Onstage they creatively express their sexuality, beauty of the body as an art form in motion and God's gift, independence, and being human. Some dancers parody the pretense that clothing gives. As subjects, not objects, they take advantage of the remunerative opportunity to deal with the life stresses of economics and single parenthood. Flexible schedules allow time for college or child rearing, and club patrons' paying to see their dancing enhances their self-esteem. The most stress for dancers seems to come from the stigma attached to being a stripper.

## Homosexuality

Being gay in American society has its stresses. In the United States, homosexual sodomy was outlawed at the time of the Constitution and was a crime in every state until 1962. Some states imposed criminal penalties. The AIDS epidemic engendered further stress and an outbreak of homophobia. The 1986 Supreme Court decision *Bowers v. Hardwick* held there is no constitutionally protected right for homosexuals or heterosexuals to engage in sodomy.

However, homosexuality became a tolerated deviance and a lifestyle cele-brated in popular film and theater as well as theater-arts dance. Then came a landmark decision in 2003. In *Lawrence v. Texas* the Supreme Court struck down the Texas ban on private consensual sex between adult homosexuals. Thirteen states had laws similar to that of Texas. Gay people are now treated equally under the law and are no longer subject to demeaning criminality and reflexive assumption of inferiority. New respect for gays will positively affect their child-custody, visitation, and adoption opportunities. There may be a decline in the stigma of the association of dance with homosexuality.

Lesbians in the past were not subject to the stress of being homosexual so much as being women. There were not court cases against them as there were against gay men.[15] Thus their danced exploration of lesbian themes is less prevalent or obvious than gays working through homosexual issues on stage.

On the fringe of society and receptive to the unconventional, the art world has long offered homosexuals a vehicle to express an aesthetic sensibility that is emotional and erotic, an insulation from a rejecting society, an avenue of courtship, and an arena in which to deal with homosexual concerns and resist, reduce, and escape stress.

Choreographic motifs about homosexuality run the gamut from unhappy to joyous, masked to unmasked, lust to love, and real gender to desired gender. Dance has captured the history of gays as a perceived public menace, symbol of death, and corruption of the soul. *Monument for a Dead Boy*, choreographed by Rudi van Dantzig in 1965, was one of the first ballets to treat the making, life, and death of a homosexual. Parents, friends, sexual encounters, and psychic trauma are displayed in fragmentary danced narrative. "The boy, it seems, has been traumatized by a brutal display of parental coitus. He can't make it with a snaky seductress in blue; he feels dirty just thinking about it. He wants to go back to the days when he kissed a little girl among the hollyhocks, but this innocence is irretrievable and he turns to a young man for comfort. For this, the boy is taunted and gang-raped by a pack of school chums. With insult heaped upon injury, the boy kills himself."[16] During the 1970s there were a number of ballets with *pas de deux* (or *trois*) for men as part of a larger work that showed the acceptance and beauty of homosexuality. For example, in *The Goldberg Variations* by Jerome Robbins, two boys dance together as two girls watch. Robbins hints at differing ways of love. *Weewis*, choreographed by Margo Sappington for the Joffrey Ballet, had a homoerotic male *pas de deux* that was about her husband's relationship with his best friend.

Some ballets are essentially homoerotic but pretend to be something else. Implicitly homosexual, Gerald Arpino's *The Relativity of Icarus* created a hulla-baloo although he denied the homosexual inference. Two male leads represent the mythic airborne figures of Daedalus and Icarus. Nearly naked, they touch each other erotically in a cantilevered duet. Although they are supposed to be father and son, audience members see no discrepancy discernible in age—which would be easily achieved by makeup, costume, and movement—to make this believable.

Lar Lubovitch has said that AIDS was the motivation for his *Concerto Six Twenty-two*, "because so many dancers have been stricken with AIDS, something the dance world doesn't own up to. . . . I felt that I wanted to show a version of male love on a platonic and high-minded level, to show the dignity of men who love each other as friends, that all men do have another man in their lives that they love so dearly, not in a homosexual relationship, but just all men."[17]

The AIDS epidemic beginning in the 1980s led to a rise in images of pain and grieving. In 1988 charismatic dancer/choreographer Bill T. Jones lost his partner and lover, Arnie Zane, to AIDS. Other friends and colleagues were succumbing. Jone created a series of intensely emotional pieces. After Zane's death, several of Jones's new dances confronted the suffering of AIDS; in one performance, he even had one of his Bill T. Jones/Arnie Zane and Company dancers who had AIDS participate in a dance even though pain prevented him from standing on his own. *La Grande Fête* and *Absence* transmitted Jones's sense of loss, mourning, mortality, and coping. In public celebration of Zane, Jones depicts the joy dance can represent in a grieving world; choreography is the medium he uses to confront his feelings and explore the struggle to survive and grow from the experience. He is HIV positive. *D-Man in the Waters* was dedicated to one of his dancers, Demian Acquavella, who was HIV positive and struggling with his health, "out there swimming, just like I'd seen Arnie swim, fighting the waters. That was the metaphor."[18] The underlying theme is individuals finding strength in struggle and in a supportive community. In fact, the whole company contributed to the choreography in a triumphant journey. Dance commemorates loved ones and ensures that loved ones are not forgotten, and that their spirit or work continues. Company members reported that the dances enabled them to better manage the situation of pain and anguish of loss caused by AIDS.

David Gere, a gay critic and academic, makes this argument: Gay choreographers use symbols from the hospital and the street, subtle and unabashed depictions of gayness, marginalization, and male-male eros to portray suffering, grieving, and mourning, as well as to celebrate and thus to lessen aches. Seeking to cope with the grisly deaths from AIDS, gay choreographers have sought to replace mainstream notions of heaven in the image of sexual ecstasy "based on the importance of penetration in gay male sexual practices of the early 1980s, and on the heightened physical sensations facilitated by arousal of prostate, anus, and penis together."[19] Eroticism is a means to metamorphose continuity of life.

## Transvestites

Transvestite dancing, long a component of the gay demimonde, surfaced from the semisecret underground of clubs, largely frequented by homosexuals, to the stages of major theaters of the world's capitals, where drag ballet has played to standing-room-only crowds. For example, Les Ballets Trockadero de Monte Carlo has been a box-office success throughout the United.States. The drag act has been called misogynist. To wit: Janice Raymond asserts that "all transsexuals rape women's bodies by reducing the real female form to an artifact, appropriating this body for themselves."[20] Yet most critics recognize the company as lovingly parodying dance conventions. Men show that they can do the same things that women can do in ballet and at the same time make a critical comment on what they should do.

Drag dance, like gay dance in general, may be a means to cope with stress by gaining public approbation in dance performance. Psychologists have pointed out that the pressure for a man to perform aggressively in a male role may be the cause for cross-dressing and related behavior.[21] In Western culture it is more acceptable for a woman to be like a man than the reverse. Transvestism recognizes the feminine element in every man's nature and acknowledges that the difference between men and women is not so great. Transvestism may thus reduce stress, create excitement, and relieve the pressure of sex-role conformity. Sometimes a caricature of the image of the opposite sex is an attempt to demonstrate the right not to adopt an essentially heterosexual way of life; the parody calls attention to the cultural blueprint and the frequency with which it is disregarded. By being a lie, the duplicity of transvestism is also a mockery of preexisting sex roles.

## Humor

Humorous dance often provides relief from stress, evoking a smile, belly laugh, or gasp of disbelief. Impersonations using the juxtaposition of a male body performing dainty feminine movements are often funny. The dancers in all-male companies tell the same joke over and over. They parody the act of performance, specific ballets, and particular styles through dance-informed in-jokes. A sturdy man struggling to cope with steps that ballet tradition has reserved for thin women creates absurdity. The ugly sisters are danced by Washington Ballet men in Septime Webre's *Cinderella*. The more serious the men are in drag, on pointe (tip of toe shoe), and in tutus, the funnier the performance. While males spoofing women is funny, the reverse is not. It's an issue of gravity; a heavy person trying to become light is automatically funnier than a light person trying to become heavy.

Humor can come from breaking rules. A highly codified form with established expectations, ballet lends itself to humor. Yet ballet is minimally funny because it has had to fight to be taken seriously. August Bournonville's *Konservatoriet* reproduces a ballet class that builds from simple steps and basic ballet positions to more-complex moves in the style of the French eighteenth-century ballet. Student mistakes are comic. Role reversal and gender blurring, women tossing and catching men, often get a laugh.

The shock of the unexpected and incongruity within a dance genre creates comic pieces. Accenting the offbeat, abrupt changes of tempo; disharmonious use of body parts; illogical cause and effect; sudden switch of movement styles; uneven meters that result in a one-sided or limping effect; and taking gestures and movements belonging to one context, such as a church, and placing them in another, such as a brothel, create humor. Satirical references to topical personalities or character types and double entendres evoke a smile. We laugh when we see ourselves and familiar situations as ridiculous.

An example of rule breaking comes from modern-dance choreographer Twyla Tharp's *Push Comes to Shove*. Danseur Mikhail Baryshnikov and his partner embrace as in classical ballet, but incongruously his feet move rapidly, violating ballet convention. In a lyric move, he picks up his partner and shakes her, an unacceptable dance act, and then they resume their lyrical expression. The dancers effortlessly move from classical ballet to Tharp's quirky style to pedestrian movement.

Jerome Robbins's *The Concert* is a sequence of sketches about audience members' fanciful daydreaming and incongruities. A motley group attends a classical-music concert. While they listen to a recital of pieces by Chopin, their mental images are embodied in dance. A girl arises and violently whirls herself into collapse. Butterflies emerge when the *Butterfly Etude* is heard. A woman tries to kill her husband. Modern-dance choreographer Paul Taylor's *Cloven Kingdom* satirizes men, who are portrayed like animals. They dangle pawlike hands, grunt, and thrash about.

Ludovic Jolivet in *Within* portrays with the comic poignancy of Charlie Chaplin the inner struggle between a man's dream, his nature, and what the capitalist system expects from him. Dressed in a suit, he grasps his briefcase. It

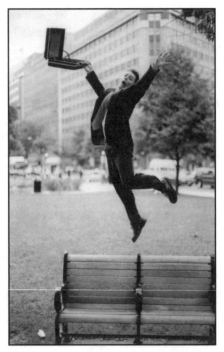

**Figure 8.11.** *Within* **(Photo of Ludovic Jolivet, City Dance, by Paul Gordon Emerson)**

tosses him this way and that. Then he's flying in dollar bills, perhaps dreaming of being in an adult entertainment exotic dance club and tipping beautiful strippers.

## Afterword

Although some dance participants perceive theatrical performance merely as entertainment and, consequently, a means to temporarily escape stress, dance has even greater potential. Through the performance of themes related to a frequently uncaring world riddled with injustice, dance may be a means to resist or reduce stress. Audience members may bear witness to a dancer's authentic anger or mourning, the release of energy mobilized in the fight-flight stress response. Choreographers, dancers, and observers may resist stress by anticipating possibilities, as described in chapter 5. Themes of death, sexuality, gender roles, violation of societal norms, discrimination, and oppression are held up to scrutiny. The nonverbal realistic or abstract storytelling of dance about stressful issues may provide catharsis for dancer and spectator and thus reduce stress. Impulses toward attraction of the forbidden may find satisfaction in fantasy. Participants in the theatrical event of dance performance may gain distance and insight that move them to resolve some of their problems. Alternatively, the themes portrayed in dance may scrape against raw nerves and induce stress.

∼

## CHAPTER NINE

# A Dance Career in the West

Most professional ballet dancers love their work and find it gratifying and empowering. Total immersion is blissful.

> Classical ballet dancers must study from the age of eight for 10 years before they might—just might—move in a way that is interesting and beautiful to watch. As professionals we work 12 hours a day for six days a week. We inhabit an environment of order, routine, discipline, beauty and youth. Our obsessive preoccupation with physical perfection is the external result of a deep, silent, and very private spiritual commitment.[1]

Thus wrote Toni Bentley who danced with New York City Ballet, one of the world's most prestigious dance organizations. Her remarks about a demanding career were in response to the suicide of a friend and colleague in the dance company. The road to becoming a professional is filled with stressors. There is no guarantee of success, even after a dancer invests a huge amount of time, effort, and money in training, self-discipline, and sacrifice. And among those who make it to the top, not all can cope with the demands of the field and their aspirations in or outside it.[2]

Film director Robert Altman spent time with the Joffrey Ballet of Chicago in order to prepare *Company*, a fictionalized documentary. Groping for words to describe the lives of the dancers he came to know and admire, he remarks, "They're so in—like—in a tube...having isolated themselves socially because the disciplines are so demanding and unique. They never make any money. They compete for very few jobs. And even when they succeed: by

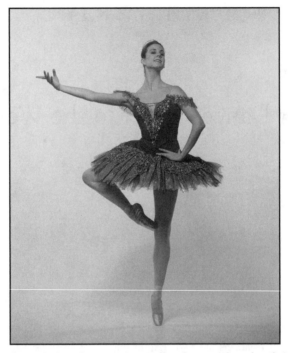

**Figure 9.1.   Michele Wiles, American Ballet Theatre (Photo by Chris Dame)**

age 34, 'fshhhht,' they're finished. . . . But they picked a very hard row to hoe, and they're out there hoeing it."[3] Producer and star Neve Campbell wanted to make the film because dance is the most unappreciated art form, and she wanted to portray the individual and collective struggle behind what appears to the audience as an effortless performance.[4]

Yet not all forms of professional dance are so demanding. For example, modern dance, jazz, and flamenco are more forgiving concerning weight, 180-degree turnout, and musculoskeletal characteristics that favor extensive pointe work. Besides dance companies, there are other performance venues such as Broadway, cruise ships, nightclubs, theme parks, live pop-music acts, TV films and music videos, schools, community institutions, and industrials (conventions and conferences at which dance routines are used to market everything from computers to shoes).

All jobs have stresses—bad bosses, unfulfilled expectations, and so on. The stresses of a professional dance career are similar to those of professional athletes.[5] Unlike most professional athletes, people today usually go into professional dance out of a passion, a calling, not for the rewards of financial security and stability, the benefits of most conventional occupations. Selfless dedication has an affinity to gift giving. Motivation to dance professionally often includes the satisfaction of achieving what others want to do, try to do, but cannot do well, and the exhilaration of performance. Dancers may perform for others and in place of others. Performance tends to catapult the successful dancer to heights of exhilaration, like the runner's high or what other athletes, astronauts, or race-car drivers experience. Many dancers seek out stress and thrive on risk and the rewards of surviving it.

Despite its stresses, a dance career may also create illusionary worlds, provide an escape from the everyday world's stresses, and offer an outlet for releasing tension. For renowned prima ballerina Gelsey Kirkland, who danced with New York City Ballet and then American Ballet Theatre, dance offered a convenient way to avoid her father, a writer who had fallen upon difficult times and had turned to alcoholism, and family fights. In her autobiography, *Dancing on My Grave* she says escaping from home to ballet also offered her a creative arena in which to vent her rage at being unable to control her home environment. "By devoting myself to the discipline of dance, I was able to establish a measure of control that was otherwise lacking in my life."[6] She was bound to the feelings and ideas that came with each breakthrough in her understanding.[7]

Attitudes toward the dancer, career development and career transition, performance anxiety, cooperation and competition, injuries, food and weight, and economic survival are some of the stressors associated with becoming and being a professional dancer. Going from one's studio as a big fish in a small pond to a company of big fish can be stressful. So, too, is hitting a plateau in artistic growth after advancing. Performers frequently need a second job when the dance company paycheck doesn't cover their bills. The company's lack of understanding about second job schedules can create stress as can getting little rest and switching mental gears. Responses to these stressors may include releasing pent-up energy; creating new forms of dance, such as modern dance and contact improvisation engaging in contemplative creativity; and seeking therapy (see chapter 11).

## Society's Attitudes toward Dancers

Twenty-six years prior to Duell's unexpected death, Agnes de Mille, renowned dancer and choreographer, drew upon a lifetime spent in the classroom, rehearsal hall, and theater to write a candid book called *To a Young Dancer: A Handbook for Dance Students, Parents, and Teachers.* De Mille noted a half century ago that dancers have always moved in "an aura curious and provocative if often at the same time despised" by some religious people who disdain all dance. Dancers, she said

> are looked upon with all the doubts visited on any vagabond. Parents would certainly hesitate about permitting a daughter to marry a dancer, while the thought of a son embracing the profession causes such acute dismay as has on occasion resulted in outright disinheritance. There is still a general reluctance to ask dancers into nice homes except on the most transient basis and prompted by curiosity.[8]

Yet De Mille recognized the presence of a continuing trend: Dancers' appeal seems popular, and their pictures appear constantly in advertising.[9]

Until the mid-twentieth century, in Europe and in the United States, dance was not considered a proper, respectable profession for ladies and gentlemen. However, working-class youth welcomed the training, livelihood, pension, and opportunity for glory. In the minds of the general public, female dancing was associated with moral laxity; male dancing has been similarly associated with moral laxity, especially homosexuality. Despite the receptivity of the art world to deviance from what is generally accepted in the broader society, some dancers made efforts to keep their sexual lives private. Many artists, such as Degas, fixated on the dancers (the good-time girls or prostitutes) of the decadent music halls of the 1890s. The attribution of immorality to dance continues up through the striptease nude dancing of the twenty-first century.[10] Although this adult entertainment is said by some to exploit women, most dancers feel stressed by the stigma expressed by mainstream society.

The disdained ballet began gaining a more respectable status in America, due partly to a decrease in the influence of puritanism and the American appearance of Serge Diaghilev's superb dancers and choreographers in 1916. The advent of modern dance in the 1920s, pioneered by educated middle-class women of strong character (such as Ruth St. Denis and Martha Graham, both of whose parents trained in medicine), and the creation of university dance programs (the University of Wisconsin in 1926 was the first) sowed the seeds to make a dance career respectable for women. Still, modern dancer Anna Sokolow, renowned in the United States, Mexico, and Israel, said that in the 1920s her mother did not approve of dancers. She asked in Yiddish, "So you're going to be a *kurve* [whore]?" "No, Mama," Sokolow replied. "I'm going to be a dancer." Her mother told her to leave the house. And so she left.[11]

A dance career for men was certainly regarded as questionable. Lincoln Kirstein, cofounder with George Balanchine of the School of American Ballet and the New York City Ballet, of which he was general director, says,

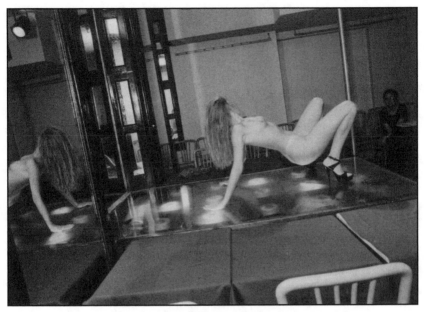

Figure 9.2. Exotic Dancer (Photo by Chris Dame)

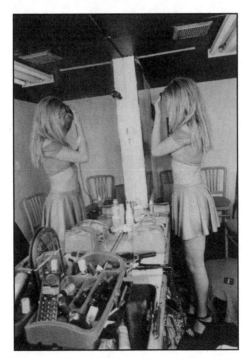

Figure 9.3. Exotic Dancer (Photo by Chris Dame)

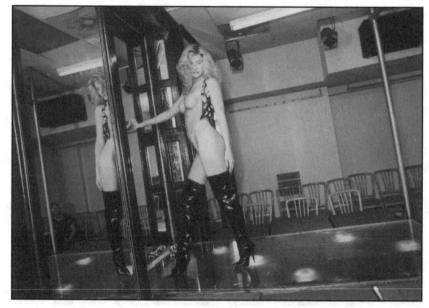

**Figure 9.4.    Exotic Dancer (Photo by Chris Dame)**

"When I grew up, a father would rather see his son dead than a dancer."[12] Choreographer Brian Macdonald said his family wanted him to be a lawyer, and his refusal was tantamount to prompt disinheritance: "The day I joined the National Ballet of Canada in 1951, my father changed his will. He died without ever changing it back."[13] Of a younger generation, Douglas Dunn, dancer/choreographer who was educated in art history at Princeton University, said his parents, both doctors, were not happy with his career choice. A 1980 pulse reading on attitudes toward dance came from Ronald Reagan's campaign headquarters: the politicians concerned with reactions of the Moral Majority seemed embarrassed that, as the *Washington Post* put it, "While his dad does the White House waltz, Ronald P. Reagan, 22, is jete-ing for the Joffrey II Dancers."[14]

Because male dancers have been assumed to be gay, they often experience persecution and torment from an early age. Rhee Gold was preparing an outstanding fifteen-year-old male dancer for an interview in a dance competition. Gold asked him what his male friends thought about his dancing (he had trained with a particular teacher since the age of three).

> All of a sudden there was silence. His confidence level went from one hundred to one. At first he started to ramble without really answering the question, so I asked it again. Within seconds, he was crying. He started telling me that he

didn't want to go to school anymore because he was constantly being harassed and he was actually beaten up several times because he danced. He said his classmates, boys and girls alike, were always calling him a fag. He was dealing with this day in and day out, and it had obviously had a major emotional effect on him.[15]

Ballet student, teacher, and anthropologist Daniel O'Connor has observed that when a male dancer (straight or gay) is among gays, he might first acknowledge the stereotypical image of the gay dancer and then establish himself as an exception. He does this by revealing, for example, that he has a girlfriend, he finds gays disgusting, or his love of ballet makes him "put up" with gay men. Another strategy is dressing like a successful businessman or gentlemanly scholar and communicating machismo through body language. Despite these stereotypes, danseur Rudolf Nureyev's and other male stars' six-digit incomes, films about macho male dancers, ballet training for athletes, and the popularity of hip-hop and jazz have spurred some measure of respectability for men in dance.

Males or females who go into the dance profession as part of an effort to enhance self-esteem (related to a faulty body image and a continuing reenactment of approach-avoidance relationships with a parental figure) may experience stress if they come from or work in a milieu in which a negative stigma is associated with dance. This paradoxically lowers self-esteem. The dancer partially fulfills a need for public approval through a process that simultaneously exacerbates that same need.[16]

Female dancers, like other working women, desire to achieve and at the same time may fear disapproval for achieving. Some struggle to compete in the workplace with men while simultaneously fulfilling the role of wife and mother.[17] Choreographer/dancer Blondell Cummings spoke at the Dance Theater Workshop's 1986 seminar about the conflict she experienced between her strict religious upbringing and the demands of her art. She had been asked to bare her chest, a violation of the biblical dictate for women to be modest.

Barriers to the acceptance of dance as a career are falling due to developments that contribute to upgrading the status of dancers and destigmatizing the profession. University dance programs, comparisons of dancers to athletes, the involvement of a range of occupational groups in dance (including policemen, as seen in televised performances staged by former New York City Ballet principal Jacques d'Amboise), and famous dancers' six-figure incomes help to overcome the reservations people have about dancers. Performers like Rudolf Nureyev, Mikhail Baryshnikov, Natalia Makarova, Alicia Alonso, Carlos Acosta, and Savion Glover are celebrities and are respected. Young

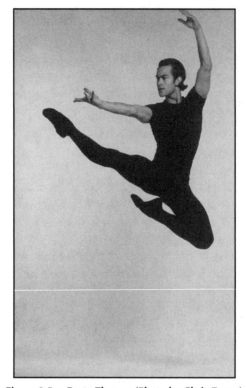

**Figure 9.5.   Rasta Thomas (Photo by Chris Dame)**

dancers—such as Rasta Thomas, who has won gold medals in international dance as well as martial arts competitions and has performed internationally as a guest artist and in dance companies and on television, film, and Broadway—are also gaining broad recognition and acceptance.[18]

## Politics

Prior to desegregation, segregation and the exclusion of African Americans from white theaters and dance companies were stressful. Black dancers had to black-up like white minstrels playing Negroes and say they were white to get performance opportunities in mainstream society. The white minstrel shows mastered and mocked African American expressive styles of performance. Moreover, blacks had to pass as whites to enter white clubs to see all-black shows intended for whites. Even after desegregation, there was a widespread assumption that the Euro-American body was better suited for ballet, and even

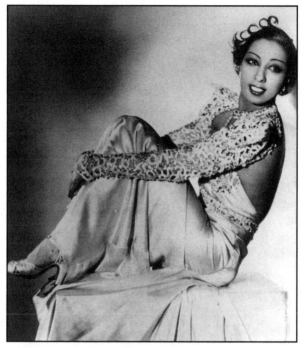

**Figure 9.6.** Josephine Baker (Photo courtesy of Jerry Murbach, www.doctormacro.com)

black spirituals, than the African American body. Only African-style dance was thought to be appropriate for blacks. Delores Browne (principal dancer in New York Negro Ballet from 1956 to 1959) has asked, "Why is it not possible for a major company to take a number of black dancers in the corps de ballet and allow them to grow up in the ensemble as anyone else would have a chance to do?"[19] She noted that the New York City Ballet had 125 dancers: "Do you really believe that there are not at least five good black female dancers in this whole nation?"[20] Raven Wilkinson, an African American dancer who passed for white, did perform with Ballet Russe de Monte Carlo and in Europe.

Josephine Baker, Arthur Mitchell, Katherine Dunham,[21] and Alvin Ailey[22] paved the way for African American dancers. For example, under George Balanchine's wing, Mitchell became in 1955 the first African American male to be a permanent member of a major ballet company, namely, New York City Ballet. Balanchine supported Mitchell's establishment of the multidimensional Dance Theatre of Harlem in 1969 and gave him great ballets to stage. Shortly after Reverend Martin Luther King Jr.'s assassination, Mitchell was inspired to establish a school that would offer youngsters—especially those in Harlem, where he was born—the opportunity to learn about dance and the allied arts. Opening a school in a Harlem garage in 1969 was his corrective for the riots he'd experienced as a boy there in the 1940s.

In 1958, Alvin Ailey founded the Alvin Ailey American Dance Theater, a highly successful modern-dance company. He drew upon the black experience in church and the jazz world for many of his dances.

Politics exists in the dance world as in any other. Students or performers may be the butt of bias, victim of favoritism, accused of disloyalty, or object of intrigue by someone's pursuit of self-advancement. Sometimes company board members or government officials interfere in artistic decision making. These situations may create stress. An individual who feels mistreated might seek a neutral person to help assess the situation, make suggestions, or try to remedy the stressor.

The renowned ballerina Anastasia Volochkova made worldwide news when the Bolshoi Ballet dismissed her for allegedly being too big and fat to be partnered. A tall, thin woman whom I observed surviving on yogurt over a two-week period when she came to the United States to have Vladimir Angelov create solo ballets for her, she was obviously involved in a political cross fire. When she was a star at the Kirov Ballet, there had been no problem in partnering her. Russia's Labor Ministry said the dancer's firing violated Russian labor laws and called on the Bolshoi to reinstate her. The Bolshoi complied

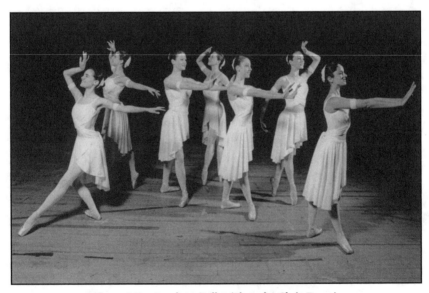

**Figure 9.7. Loudoun Ballet (Photo by Chris Dame)**

but did not give her the major roles she had had. So Volochkova filed suit against the Bolshoi Ballet. "Unfortunately, I have to do it because I am seeking justice and want to assert my rights as well as the rights of other artists."[23]

## Choreographers and Dance-Company Managers Challenge Dancers

Irrespective of government or private funding of dance, the choreographer/ artistic director often has absolute creative control and considers the dancer an expendable commodity. Enforced infantilism and disregard for dancers' physical and psychological well-being and personal lives are stressful. Ron Reagan, explaining why he quit the ballet, pointed out that dancers are "willing slaves to an art in which management calls the shots and holds their contracts," and dancers "must tolerate verbal abuse and ridicule."[24]

Ballet dancer Gary Chryst noted that a choreographer knows a person at eighteen and then the person is not eighteen any more and expects to be treated differently, yet still needs direction and correction.[25] Richard Le Blond Jr., former president of the San Francisco Ballet, takes up the point: "Perhaps dancers live in a world where they're not permitted to reach emotional maturity, and that really comes out in the language itself. What other profession calls adult artists 'kids'? What other profession refers to people who have been practitioners of their art and [are] in their thirties as 'boys' and 'girls'?"[26]

Gelsey Kirkland and Suzanne Farrell have contrasting perspectives on working with Balanchine.[27] Farrell was Balanchine's legendary muse, a goddess-like inspiration. They had great love for each other, but their forty-plus-year disparity in age and Balanchine's marriage at the time led Farrell to center their relationship on ballet. Balanchine had married five of his muses. The "elusive muse" and ballet maker displayed their love most poignantly in dance making in the studio and onstage. About the dances he created for her, Farrell says, "I learned to dance differently than I would have if I had had to imitate the movements of other women—I had more freedom, more choices, and less pressure to duplicate . . . unable to see the movement on any other body but Balanchine's, I had to invent my own way of moving—like him, but like a woman on *pointe* as well."[28]

Together they experimented. Balanchine wanted Farrell to be "off-balance," one of the most unorthodox requests any well-trained ballet master could make. In *Don Quixote* we "broke one rule after the other and climbed through the walls of balletic convention to discover a whole new place to inhabit . . . a tilted, revolving circle," Farrell remarks.[29]

But Kirkland says Balanchine "assembled steps that were supposed to have been predetermined by God and humbly described himself as an instrument of divine will. His word was holy."[30] Moreover, "he sought to replace personality with his abstract ideal of physical movement. . . . The interpretive stamp of a dancer threatened to mar the choreographic design of the master. . . . The master was not to be questioned. His dictum was 'Just dance.'"[31] Although Balanchine was famous for describing ballet as "Woman," because it was the ballerina who inspired him, Kirkland perceived that an inspired approach to dancing for his dancers was almost unthinkable. "He often said, 'There is no such thing as inspiration.' Our devotion made us dependent on him for ideas and psychological motivation."[32]

According to the aesthetic code of Balanchine and his collaborator, the composer Stravinsky, "the human condition was reflected primarily through animal and mechanical imagery, to be realized through the senses by way of instinct and imitation. . . . Stravinsky put it, 'An artist is simply a kind of pig snouting truffles.'"[33]

Obviously, enforced infantilism creates stress for thinking dancers. Free discussion is supplanted by idol worship and prejudice. Kirkland says, "The difficulty with Balanchine, as with many of the Russian men I have known, was that he did not think women were capable of engaging him with ideas."[34] Yet "I knew that my dance was both an act of will and a means of expression. Ballet was the only link that I had ever been able to make between thought and action."[35]

Kirkland had a zeal for perfection, yet she was filled with passivity and guilt instilled by the ballet culture. She feared to challenge the prevailing aesthetic and popular authority figures. Rage festered inside her.[36] When she felt like a failure, she tried to reassert control. "I began to starve myself . . . I was trying to disappear, to deny my physical existence altogether . . . I wanted to empty myself out completely. Purification and punishment seemed to go hand in hand."[37] Ultimately, the stress of the milieu that demanded unquestioning conformity led Kirkland to further self-destructive behavior: taking cocaine to be able to work and dance in a theater that "rejected perfection in favor of expediency and box office receipts."[38]

Balanchine did not like his female dancers dating; he wanted their sole devotion. "Motivated more by jealousy than concern, Balanchine encouraged an atmosphere that was a mixture of convent and harem."[39] To be sure, dance sometimes siphoned off sexual energies. However, the permissive attitudes of the times were at odds with the discipline of dance and its spartan work ethic. Kirkland writes: "Under the strictures imposed by Balanchine, sex was about the only weapon his dancers possessed. Defying the sexual taboo makes it seem possible to escape his domination."[40]

Directors and managers often do not regard the dancers as humans subject to physical and mental trauma in spite of their high energy and resilience. Kirstein compares the excitement of ballet to the excitement of battle and its physical risks. "Dancers are always at hazard, always in an extreme situation. When your body is in danger, it illuminates a whole other capacity. It gives you new muscle. It throws you back on yourself."[41]

Although Balanchine recognized children's physical vulnerability, "in actual practice," claims Kirkland, "his teachers unwittingly encouraged young dancers to self-destruct, rationalized as part of the sacrifice that must be made to the art. The speed and shortcuts that he built into the training process called for physical cheating in which the dancer distorted the body to deliver the position or step that Balanchine demanded. . . . I watched many of my friends become casualties and fall by the wayside."[42] Balanchine's insensitivity toward the dancer appears in his own words: "Dear, you're young. Young people don't have injuries. Go home and read fairy tales. Try little red wine . . . you need nothing but this place. You don't need anybody else. . . . You have a beautiful theater here. You come in the morning. When you don't work, you go into studio by yourself; you do *relevés* [raising the body on the ball of the foot or on the toes]. You must stay here all day; you go home. . . . That's all you need."[43] On tour with the New York City Ballet, Kirkland became emaciated, green, and seriously ill in Moscow. Balanchine insisted she perform. She had no replacement, it was opening night, and there were important people in the audience. Balanchine gave her a "vitamin" so that she would "feel much better."[44]

Farrell takes exception with Kirkland's assertion that Balanchine's training is harmful. Farrell thinks it in no way contributed to her hip problem (deterioration required hip replacement and ended her dancing career). "I think his technique preserved my body and its abilities far longer than might have been expected. It is to the speed, musicality, and consistency of his training and the freedom of adaptability it allows that I attribute my ability to dance for three years in spite of a deteriorating hip. His training in no way threatened or destroyed the human body."[45]

Because of the pervasiveness of stressful relationships between choreographers and dancers, the Dancers Forum came into being. It is a group dedicated to the improvement of the working life of dancers that began in 1996 with Dance Theater Workshop's retreats for dancers, choreographers, and presenters. In 2002 the Dancers Forum published its deliberations, *The Dancers Forum Compact for a Working Artistic Relationship between Dancers and Choreographers*, a guide that offers recommendations for both apprentice professional dancers and includes topics that give clues to the dance world: points of discussion between dancer and choreographer: methods of communication, expectations, working conditions, schedules, compensation, fringe benefits, medical expenses, reimbursements, travel, safety, appearance, discrimination, and harassment. A commentary explores rehearsal needs and conditions, attendance policy, breaks, warm-up and cool-down, and etiquette. Performance repertory and casting, performance-rehearsal-tech schedule, engagement logistics, education and publicity, complementary and discount tickets, and pre- and post-performance cleanup are addressed. In addition, the discussion of touring includes itinerary, residency activity, work on travel days, days off, transportation, travel reimbursement, housing, food and health, and meetings. Evaluation and approaches to conflict resolution are also concerns covered in the publication. The Dancers Forum hopes to stimulate creative problem solving and to foster solutions not yet envisioned by the authors. The working agreement between dancer and choreographer tends to be unique to each situation.

Of course, there are many choreographers who deviate from traditional authoritarian patterns and make dances with their dancers. It is common for choreographers to choose an idea and ask company members to express it in movement improvisation. From these movements and phrases, the choreographer then develops a work. Some companies, like Pilobolus, create dances through the interactions of company members as equals.

Some dance companies, especially smaller ones, have support networks. Mitch Allen, a professional dancer for two decades (with, among other companies, the Aman Folk Ensemble), told me, "Every dance company I've ever belonged to has become like family, where the individual's personal, physical, and professional issues are addressed by company members. The group helps buffer the stress of the profession and related life issues."

## Improvisation Movement and Contemplative Creativity

The stress of having to conform to a particular dance style and its related training and professional practices often catalyzes new movements and genres. For example, unhappiness with the structure of the ballet world and what it represents, its male dominance, traditional movement dictates, training requirements, choreography, performance, and production have provoked the "modern" dance rebellion of Isadora Duncan, Loie Fuller, and successive generations of modern dancers. In modern dance, individuals often would work with a company and then strike out on their own, such as

Erik Hawkins, who danced (and married) and then broke away from Martha Graham to develop a more relaxed, natural style of dance. Dissatisfaction with modern dance led to the genre generally labeled postmodern dance.

Contact improvisation, which refers to movements or choreographic decisions not fully set before they are performed, is in a sense a reaction to the three above-mentioned dance genres. Improvisation participation is a way to resist and reduce the stress of hierarchical teacher-student relationships, being collectively molded to an authoritative ideal of a particular dance style, and the stratified performance star system. The contact-improvisation movement's egalitarian nature and allowance for individuality, a strong tradition beginning with modern dance, was a key attraction for participants.[46] Some appreciate the noncompetitive atmosphere in which individuals play with one another, a contrast with the usual pattern of student competition for teacher attention and approval. Improvisation is a way of freeing yourself from set movement patterns and erasing some of the imprints of traditional dance technique as well as differentiating yourself from a teacher or a tradition.

Moreover, the improvisation in which participants engage in an activity requiring communal group experience of unpredictable cooperative and egalitarian interactions allows the experience of self-awareness and self-discovery as a person and not just as a dancer. Trust is essential for dancers, who touch each other and bear each other's weight. Improvisers thus see dance as a transforming experience. In these ways, contact improvisation incorporates elements of dance therapy (chapter 11). An audience can identify with the process of the dancer's immediate decision making, creativity, and trust.

Improvisation is a prominent practice at the Dance/Movement Studies Department of the Naropa Institute in Boulder, Colorado. Here it is combined with "sitting contemplation" (which involves "coming to stillness" and ultimately "connecting directly with the raw energy of the phenomenal world") and contemplative choreography.[47] Naropa philosophy and practice derive from the Buddhist tradition of *shamatha/vipashyana*, or mindfulness/awareness practice. Barbara Dilley, a former performer with the postmodern Merce Cunningham Company, the Judson Dance Theatre, and Grand Union in New York City says:

> I was interested in what it would be like for other dancers to slow down and work with training their minds. I wanted to help them peel away the unnecessary aspects of their training and become more basic, more fundamental. It is not that I wanted to throw out the American dance tradition. It seems there is an aspect of the American creative process that is genuine and clear; but then there is another aspect that is highly neurotic, escapist, and fundamentally aggressive. I wanted to start at the beginning, and then sort it out from there.[48]

## Performance Anxiety, Cooperation, and Competition

A dancer's life is one of continual competition, cooperation, and performance. Training itself is a kind of performance. Students compete for the teacher's attention and approval.[49] Teachers compete for students. Dancer Rasta Thomas says students who want exposure to a variety of dance styles often face possessive dance teachers who want exclusivity. "They want you under their wing."[50]

Dancers always depend on others' evaluations: teachers; judges at schools, auditions, and other competitions; choreographers who select dancers for special roles; and audiences, including those special members, the critics.[51] Competitions are controversial and stressful. Students with fragile egos and shaky self-esteem may take the competitions personally and suffer when they lose. A second-place winner in one competition threw his trophy in the garbage can![52]

Yet competitions also have benefits. Many organizations not only provide opportunities for competition but they offer students the opportunity to take dance classes with various teachers to advance their knowledge and skill and expose them to different forms and styles of dance. Thomas, who has won over one hundred competitions, described to me how the competitions helped him. "Competitions motivated hard work. . . . Competing helps bring out the character inside you. It gives you good stage presence. Judges are there to help you, give criticism. Some important people come to you, and they introduce you to others. It's one continuing process. Besides, I like traveling and seeing the world."[53] Dance competitions have also been praised for giving young contestants a realistic perspective about their abilities in relation to their peers. Competitions can raise personal standards and give sheltered students some sense of what the real dance world is like—highly competitive and stressful. Furthermore, competitions give competitors the opportunity to win trophies, cash, and scholarships. Dance-company directors often sit in the audience scouting for performers. In a competitive society, dance competitions provide students with tangible goals. Some parents, hoping their youngster's winnings will help pay for her or his dance education and related expenses, judge a dance school by how many trophies are in the window. Many major performing and choreography competitions held worldwide every year are, in a sense, high-level auditions for places in first-rate dance companies, at prestigious dance schools, and with fine coaches.

There is always pressure, even when evaluators build up a budding talent with positive feedback. Expectations for high standards and perfectionism cannot always be met. Victoria Bromberg of the New York City Ballet reflected upon her experiences at the School of American Ballet:

> The competition at SAB wasn't necessarily a bad thing, because it prepared you for the competition and discipline in the company.... You learn how to keep yourself together.... There is no probation period in the New York City Ballet as there is in the Paris Opera, where they give you a year to pull yourself together if you let yourself get out of shape or fall down on technique.[54]

Although competitions and professional dance require performance, appearing in front of an audience can be scary.[55] Stage fright is a deviation from the person's usual level of anxiety that activates the flight-or-fight stress-response mechanism.

> Performance means being on the spot. You are "out there." You are vulnerable. You are naked. Everything shows. There is no place to hide, because even if you seek it, then that is what shows.... This is at once the magic of performance and the terror of it. It is both what attracts us to it and which induces us to make such statements as, "I will never perform again." It is our banner and our hara-kiri sword. In our times, the sense of being on edge has been heightened by two factors. One is the separation that has been created between performance and audience. It can be a paralyzing split. The second is the ethic of individuality, which produces aggression and intensifies the frozen quality of the performance arena.[56]

Dancing in front of an audience involves risk—a slip, misstep, an offbeat gesture, forgetting what is supposed to be done. Fear of failure is most troubling. Dreadful apprehension may also occur when the theme of the dance threatens to become real; that is, the roles the dancers enact are too close to the performer's immediate personal life experiences. For novices, stage appearances are frightening because they are inexperienced. Some professional dancers, however, have stage fright with anxiety attacks of jitters, sweating, shaking, feeling faint, and needing to use the toilet all their lives.[57] Paul Taylor, one of the world's great choreographers, writes in his autobiography, *Private Domain*: "Stage fright. Some clone, not me, is cowering offstage and covered with icy sweat, his palms and soles slippery, temples booming, tongue dry, seizured, sizzled. It's plain to see that the reason for greasepaint is to prevent your skin from betraying its cowardly color."[58] He at one time turned to drugs to cope.

Yet the stress of stage fright also has beneficial effects. Some excitement evokes alertness and may lead to the performer's heightened awareness, sensitivity, and drive to succeed.

Why do some dancers get nervous before a performance while others do not? The answer may lie in their training experiences. Youngsters who have a large proportion of successes develop confidence. Those who have many failures often develop expectations of further mistakes and consequently experience negative stress. Some teachers do not discuss stage fright with their young performers because they believe that fear is contagious. Others talk about it in a supportive way to reassure performers that stage fright is not unusual. Waiting until they have something to respond to, teachers avoid the risk that the student will unconsciously experience the teacher as wanting the student to experience anxiety or suffering.[59]

Admission to a conservatory requires students to audition before a group of critical people who may provide negative comments. Upon a student's graduation, jobs require auditions. That is, there is a series of events in a performance career, each with possible negative reinforcements. The negative aspect of competition may produce a bad self-image, tension, and anxiety.

In Kirkland's experience, "the vicious pressure of competition invariably turned dancer against dancer."[60] The success of one dancer may be the failure of another. Moreover, success is not something static. A dancer is continually being tested.

Bentley took her first ballet lesson at the age of three. In her journal she wrote about her School of American Ballet audition eight years later. At last her name was called, and she and her mother walked into the office. Yes, they would take this thin, graceful youngster. Thrilled by a triumph that she had not planned, she felt success for the first time, along with the realization that her success was inevitably connected with the failure of others. However, five months after her admission, the school had doubts about her talent, future, and feet. It was not certain that she would be allowed to continue after the first year. She was so angry that she threw her beloved toe shoes down the incinerator. Her parents were shocked at the apparent pain she felt.[61]

However, she succeeded in the school and during her seven years moved to the top. Others had been weeded out. Some grew too tall, fell in love, or went to college. During her last year she injured her foot and could not dance for three months. Upon her return to class, Balanchine was there to select girls to perform the ballerina parts in the school's workshop performance, the pinnacle in the student's career. He chose her to learn the role of Princess Aurora in *The Sleeping Beauty*. After six months of rehearsal, she slipped the week before the performance. Despite sitting for the last week of rehearsals in a chair with a black and blue ankle packed in ice, on the morning of the performance, she danced. She felt no pain at all but was injured for a month afterward. But she had danced, and she had triumphed. She was not going to give up the chance of a lifetime.[62]

Bentley realized her dream and joined the New York City Ballet. What is more, she was chosen for special parts. And then one day instead of seeing her name listed alone, as is the case for dancers who are selected for solos, it was seen with others. "So perhaps the road to Ballerina Land was not going to be as straight as I had planned. . . . It was devastating. The straight lines . . . zigzagged all over the place. Going forward used to mean going forward. I think now that it means going backward."[63] At the age of twenty-two, she felt dancing was not serving her purpose. "Unless you're out there on the big stage alone, you've no chance to communicate and know you're being successful."[64] Experiencing a stagnating career, she reflected:

> I suppose I should be happy I am still young enough to begin again, but I've no money, no lover, no future I can see, only the same ballets, seasons after seasons. . . . What else is there? There is the example of the good survivors, those who bounce back over and over. They have an outside life and outside interests, so when dancing fails, they can keep themselves occupied in a nondestructive way and wait for the will to dance to emerge again of its own accord.[65]

Bentley took a leave of absence from the New York City Ballet and then returned. She had to leave to see what she had left: "the bliss of total immersion, total concentration in dancing . . . I have a joy and an energy. . . . I am a dancer."[66]

Although aspiring dancers seek to study and perform in New York City, the dance capital of the United States—perhaps the world—the city has its special stresses. Sara Maule, who came from the West Coast and joined American Ballet Theatre, remembers being overwhelmed by the hugeness of everything in New York.

> San Francisco was a cosmopolitan city, but New York was still a shock. In San Francisco I had teachers who took care of me and nurtured me. What was most traumatic about New York was the anonymity. There were so many dancers, all with different reasons for being there, all going their separate ways. There were so many people in class that the teacher was more impersonal too. Joining Ballet Theatre helped. Once you're in a union company the pay is good and you have good job security. But that in itself was a shock. Ballet Theatre was such a big company—there were so many people, and everyone fighting to make it. It was a family, but after my experience in San Francisco, a big, impersonal one.[67]

When dancers are supposed to master new dance material that is markedly different from previous ways of moving, they may experience anxiety, even depression. There is also post-performance stress. The steep fall from a high of giving so much on stage, being transformed and adored, and then the curtain comes down with final bows, and it's like having to begin life over. One dancer put it this way: "After being something on stage, you're just back to you—you feel you're nothing."[68]

A continual stressor for the choreographer and dancer is the popular belief that, as David White, a dance producer puts it, "You are only as good as your last review."[69] The choreographer and dancer are treated as commodities: when talent burns out, another fresher model is waiting to star. The intensity of performances, even when dancers perform with a physical injury, has at times been heightened by artificial resources of energy.

Thomas, who trained at the Universal Academy of Ballet and became the winner of gold medals at prestigious competitions, international guest artist, and film actor/dancer, all before the age of twenty, has felt the stress of staying at the top. He went on to be the youngest Dance Theatre of Harlem principal. When the company went on hiatus, he became a star of choreographer Twyla Tharp's Broadway show *Movin' Out*.

The greatest stress in ballet, Thomas believes, is that "ballet is a perfect art on paper and in theory. And creating perfect art when you're not perfect or feeling perfect is frustrating. You battle with life, what you have for breakfast, how you wake up, how your muscles feel—every day. Coping with stress depends on the drive. Gelsey [Kirkland] and Misha [Baryishnikov] were fanatical about perfection."[70]

Choreographers, the creators of dances, may experience anxiety about being able to produce. Perfectionists worry about their work measuring up to their high standards. Pressures of deadlines and limited resources intensify the situation. Choreographers are risk takers and fear failure. They must innovate as Western aesthetics dictates. However, too much innovation can lose audiences unfamiliar with, or unreceptive to, the avant-garde. In terms of blockbusters, dance audiences are attracted to what they know—usually a classical ballet they've seen or a dance that has a familiar plot. The positive features of creators as unique and marvelous have their negative counterparts, a loner-outsider, troublemaker, uncommitted.

## Injuries

Thirty-year-old Neve Campbell speaks of her own training at Canada's National Ballet School: "I've had bunions. I've had broken toes. I've had fallen arches. I've had strained tendons in my arches. I've had tendonitis in my Achilles'. I've had torn ligaments and sprained ankles in both ankles. Shin splints. Pulled calves. In my knees, I've had chondromalacia and tendonitis. I've had pulled hamstrings. I've had snapping-hip syndrome and arthritis in my hips. I've had sciatic problems in my back and the arthritis in my neck. Oh, and I sprained my wrists." Not complaining, she explained how hard the career to which she once aspired can be.[71]

Dancers are subject to the over-use syndrome—every time they exercise their bodies, their muscles are injured, and if they exercise again before the muscles have recovered, they tear. Break dancing may cause blood vessels in the brain to break, leading to stroke. Contemporary repertoires often call for a high degree of athleticism, and dancers do not always have the cross-training needed to stay healthy.

High levels of anxiety appear to be a potent factor that leads to injuries.[72] Dancers need to manage stress from exhaustion due to efforts to achieve perfectionism and a 9 AM-to-11 PM day during which there are parts to learn, classes to take, grueling rehearsals to attend, and performances to give. Other stressors to manage are being subjected to training that dance-medicine research has found counterproductive and being fearful of speaking out, as well as the need to cope with an injury and the potential loss of roles or even a career as a dancer, forced retirement, loss of income, and identity.

Fearful that the doctor will tell them not to use an injured body part for a period of time and someone will take their place, dancers may choose not to seek help with injuries. An injured person suffers a loss of identity as a dancer, often without having a replacement identity. Self-doubt concerning recuperation or finding some other career are stressful.

Hormonal problems, poor nutrition, and residual tightness or weakness from a prior injury may occur. Too much exercise may lead to body fat declining to levels so low that the body goes into its starvation-coping mode and menstruation ceases, a condition known as amenorrhea. If this persists for five years or more, an irreversible loss of bone mass occurs making the person vulnerable to bone fractures, especially in the spine, hips, and wrists.

Dancers whose daily life is built around that high, the feeling of well-being that can come at the end of a workout or performance become psychologically addicted to this feeling. Thus they experience psychic distress when an illness comes on. Without dance activity, they may become irritable, tense, and anxious; dancers in a company fear someone else will take their roles forever, and they sometimes fall into depression, experiencing lethargy and a loss of interest in eating, sex, and other activities. Getting back to prior fitness levels may be a painful, frustrating process.

Children are vulnerable to their own kind of injury in dance. A child younger than eight years old lacks bones insufficiently strong to withstand heavy or prolonged physical discipline required by a dance career. For this reason, classes for three and four year olds have creative movement and play with elements of dance. Older children study the rudiments of a dance form.

Children may be asked by parents, teachers, or coaches to accomplish more than they are physically and emotionally ready for, resulting in stress. Age, development, and multicultural expectations affect readiness, although some youngsters are naturally precocious. Juggling such things as academic requirements and dance classes, or being unable to go to friends' parties because of class or rehearsal commitments, can also be stressful.

Some parents unhealthily attempt to realize their own romantic theatrical ambitions through their offspring. Hortensia Fonseca, a dance instructor at Maryland Youth Ballet who is closely involved in the lives of her students, told me that

> Very often parents begin to realize their youngsters have talent; they see them perform. But the parents push these children a lot. They take them to auditions and urge them to take part in school and other local shows. Sometimes the floors [at these performances] are not right for dance. The children suffer tendonitis, shin splints, and knee and back injuries. They are taken to doctors, chiropractors, and physical therapists. They drop out if there are insufficient resources for treatment. The parents don't realize their children are too young to be doing so much. I tell the parents they are not helping the children.[73]

Youngsters may also impose unrealistic demands upon themselves. Because there are now numerous sources of information, students are able to read about dance, the competitions, prizes, and scholarships—and they push themselves to obtain them. Impatient, they believe their bodies are indestructible. Body changes in puberty may lead to a youngster's body no longer being appropriate for professional ballet. "I try to calm them," says Fonseca. Furthermore, those students who attend dance-education boarding schools, which offer both dance and academics, often feel homesick.

Burnout, a condition of physical, mental, and emotional exhaustion from a person's inability to cope with the demands of dance and its stressors and consequent loss of interest in dance, may occur. This condition affects children and adults alike.

## Food and Weight

Abnormal thinness, the current reigning aesthetic for dancers of ballet and much of modern dance, contributes to health by placing less stress on vital organs during strenuous activity, to fleetness, and to a dancer's ability to be lifted easily. Eating what one likes is not always compatible with staying in shape. The competition between one's culinary desires and one's career demands create a range of stresses. Dance-studio mirrors are constant reminders of body shape.

Ballet dancers' weight is about 15 percent below what scientists consider a healthy weight. Medical doctor Douglas Anderson notes: "Ballet students collectively comprise the highest risk group for the development of serious eating disorders. The incidence of anorexia nervosa runs as high as seven percent in professional dance schools in North America and Europe."[74] The ballet-company mentality of prolonged immaturity and dependency makes dancers, who are without strong emotional support from family or authority figures, susceptible to bodily abuse. Gifted dancers who are pushed within the company are placed under persistent pressure. Companies usually accept neither the responsibility nor the financial burden of providing professional counseling and care for those dancers.

Relentless pursuit of the unnatural "ideal" female body arrests puberty, imbalances hormones, causes menstrual dysfunction, contributes to hypothermia and low blood pressure, and invites brittle bones and injury. Moreover, this pursuit often leads to psychosomatic disorders of starvation (anorexia nervosa) and vomiting and the use of laxatives (bulimia nervosa), which are interconnected with the incidence of injury.[75] These eating disorders are also misplaced efforts to control one's destiny. Ballet choreographers and directors—"almost always male—mold ballet's young women to the idea of feminine that equates beauty and grace with excessive thinness," an aesthetic that is punitive and misogynist.[76] Balanchine set the standard. Kirkland reports: "He halted class and approached me for a kind of physical inspection. With his knuckles, he thumped on my sternum and down my rib cage, clucking his tongue and remarking, 'must see the bones.' . . . He did not merely say, 'eat less.' He said repeatedly, 'Eat nothing.' "[77]

## Economic Survival

Contrary to the private enterprise nature of dance in the United States, governments in other countries often subsidize major and sometimes minor dance companies and schools. These governments maintain dancers as civil servants, and they are cared for with salaries and pensions, and respected the whole of their lives. The Soviet Union, until its dissolution; China; the United Kingdom; France; Sweden; Denmark; and Cuba are among the countries whose governments have supported dance.[78]

A persistent economic pinch is felt in the United States, where performing artists are more prone to unemployment than other members of the workforce. A 1980 study, *Employment in the Performing Arts: Reality and Myth*, by the Labor Institute for Human Enrichment, found 76 percent of professional dancers had experienced some unemployment, compared with 18 percent for other members of the workforce.[79] And because dance offers seasonal rather than full-time work, not having enough weeks of performance to be eligible for unemployment insurance is a powerful stressor. By the twenty-first century, the Rand Corporation found the situation unchanged.[80] According to John Munger of Dance USA, the range of income dancers earn is wide. Many dancers in small companies are paid poorly, irregularly, or not at all. They work as independent contractors and commonly receive an hourly flat rate of $15 per hour for rehearsals and performances or a $75 honorarium per performance. Major dance companies pay weekly salaries, $500 to $550 for corps members, $650 to $700 for soloists, $900 to $950 for principals, and $2,000 for stars. Dancers work for less than 52 weeks per year and usually without paid vacation. On tour they receive an additional allowance for room and board and extra compensation for overtime. Dancers often supplement their income by working as guest artists with other dance companies, choreographing, teaching dance, or taking jobs unrelated to the field.

The U.S. Department of Labor Bureau of Labor Statistics *Occupational Outlook Handbook 2006–07* reported that professional dancers and choreographers held somewhat more than 38,000 jobs in 2004. Median annual earnings of salaried choreographers were $33,670. The middle 50 percent earned between $21,530 and $48,940. The lowest 10 percent earned less than $14,980, and the highest 10 percent earned more than $68,190. Median annual earnings were $34,090 for choreographers working in dance studios, schools, and dance halls. Union contracts that cover various health and pension benefits alleviate some economic stress.

Rand reported that three broad trends describe the population of dancers. First, their numbers have been growing. Amateurs, unpaid dancers, are estimated to outnumber professionals by a factor of twenty or thirty to one. Second, professional dancers continue to dedicate themselves to their art despite the fact that their inflation-adjusted pay and job security have scarcely improved since the 1970s. Third, the presence of commercial-sector superstars polarizes dancers' incomes and tilts the dance career toward a select few whose wages are above everyone else's. The rare superstar earns millions of dollars annually (an estimate that likely includes salary plus income from freelance guest-artist performances and investment based on earned income), whereas the typical artist makes little more than minimum wage.

Indeed, performing-arts organizations are becoming polarized by size, whether they concentrate on so-called high art or mass entertainment. The large groups rely heavily on marketing campaigns and celebrity artists, whereas small groups focus on low-budget productions and may depend on volunteer labor, activities carried out by avocational associations, such as folk dance groups. The volunteer sector, in contrast to the nonprofit sector, relies more on contributed labor rather than monetary contributions for survival. Many of these organizations serve a particular geographic, ethnic, or cultural community.

Forecasting a fiscal siege for dance, a National Endowment for the Arts study predicts that "not-for-profit dance companies may see as much as a 30% loss of earned income in the next few years, and even a heavier fall in contributions."[81] When there is economic constriction, the arts are the first occupation to experience cutbacks. Companies hire fewer dancers, eliminate live music, spend less on costumes and set design, decrease the number of performances, and even collapse. The United States in the aftermath of 9/11 has seen dramatic cutbacks in the arts and such funding casts a lengthening shadow. Ticket sales, private giving, foundation grants, corporate donations, and state funding have shriveled. California's former $18 million arts budget was hacked to less than $2 million. Missouri eliminated its art appropriations altogether and is dipping into a cultural trust fund. Dance organizations working under tight economic constraints tend to employ hit-or-miss approaches to "participation-building."[82]

Even in one of the foremost ballet companies in the world, where dancers have steady jobs and are among the highest paid, economic survival can be a problem. Bentley says about money: "I really think we are the most ignorant paid people on earth. I'm sure we are constantly cheated and never complain. Money is only to pay for the apartment, to buy a fur coat and ballet clothes."[83] Principal dancers in New York may dole out 40 to 50 percent of their income for rent alone. Kirkland's routine of daily practice and preparation kept her broke paying for taxis to classes and rehearsals at various studios in the city; besides health clubs for swimming, whirlpool treatments, and sauna; and more-specialized facilities for massage and physical therapy. Discretionary dollars went into practice clothes, wigs, cosmetics, and a myriad of related items, including costumes whenever the need arose.[84]

Conflict between economic interests and loyalty create stress. For example, in 1980, New York City Ballet dancers and management came to a deadlock; a strike seemed imminent. Mr. B, as the dancers lovingly addressed Balanchine, when told was predictably upset and emotional. He said he would do his best, and if the dancers wanted to run the company, he would leave with his ballets.

"We are his company, his creation, his tools; without him we are nothing, and without us—well, he needs us, but he can always find dancers. The question seems rather basic: do we want to fight for our own pockets, or do we give a little for him?"[85] Many of the dancers who barely knew him, since the company had grown so large, made their stand. "They cry they have belief in him as an artist but not as their dictator. But how can one separate the two when his art can be produced only out of a state that he alone must rule? It's a pity he needs a hundred individuals as his tools rather than paintbrushes."[86]

Dance Theatre of Harlem, the highly acclaimed predominantly African American neoclassical ballet company that Arthur Mitchell, the first African American danseur in New York City Ballet, founded in 1969, was artistically successful. Nevertheless, it went into hiatus in 2004. With a deficit of $2.3 million, DTH laid off its dancers and canceled performances for the 2004–2005 season. Most dance companies were suffering from slashes in arts funding, especially following 9/11. But DTH also had a pattern of financial and administrative instability stretching back to a similar hiatus in 1990 and a chronic inability to hold on to an executive director. In addition to being artistic director, Mitchell wanted to direct the DTH business as well as to be its artistic director.

A key issue of economic survival is the conflict between needing to raise money from the public or private sector and maintaining artistic integrity in addition to finding time to create. Most dance groups depend on grants to survive, since the arts rarely pay for themselves. Many arts councils are not permitted to give money directly to artists to create new works, so dancers spend time and money to form tax-free educational foundations. Changes in funding structures and corporate sponsorships meant companies had to develop administrative structures. Economic pressures turn dance into a business. Grants often require work to be produced in certain seasons for fiscal reasons. Companies may not develop new works because administrators prefer known box-office quantities. Packaging dance to attract audiences is necessary. Then the question arises as to who owns the creative work.

Like many independent dancers/choreographers, Nejla Yatkin feels "the pressure to be constantly producing, to be visible all the time in order to get the next grant—the lifeblood and addiction of the artistic process. But dance takes time, reflection, and experimentation. The body learns much slower than the mind. It takes time to transfer a concept into the body."[87]

Although national, state, and local arts agencies' grants to dancers may be small, their grants often provide the imprimatur necessary for private funding. Peer review, the process by which artists evaluate artists, commonly selects dance proposals to fund. Stress arises when evaluators favor a particular style at a specific point in time. This may induce some conformity and compromise of aesthetic goals. To obtain grants, dancers/choreographers usually need favorable reviews from critics, and they, too, have their biases.

"The less money there is available, the higher the degree of selling," says Present Company's artistic director, Wendy Woodson. "How much can we play up to the bourgeois establishment and get money from them?"[88] She thinks there is too much business now in art, because "there is a point at which they are incompatible. It's a very delicate balance—if you are too much into making money, the purpose of doing art is diminished." What kept Woodson and her collaborator, Achim Nowak, targeted on their artistic goal was their work at community-oriented institutions. Of course, audience expectations and innovative choreography may create economic crises. Groups have to give the audience what it wants in order to attract spectators. At the same time, dancers try to stretch and brainwash the audience to accept new images.

In many parts of the United States, finding low-cost space for dance studios, rehearsal, and performance can be stressful. The problem of real-estate needs for the dance profession and other arts organizations became so severe that the New York City Department of Cultural Affairs and Office of Business Development commissioned a study of spaces for the arts within its jurisdiction.[89] There was inexpensive, suitable real estate for arts activity in abundant supply in the "valley" between the high-rise areas of Lower Manhattan and Midtown Manhattan. As older commercial and industrial structures in areas like SoHo, Tribeca, NoHo, and Chelsea lost their traditional tenants, substantial space was leased to arts organizations at low rates. Then rising rents in Midtown and Lower Manhattan caused many commercial tenants to relocate to the valley and push up rents as much as 200 to 300 percent. Between 1985 and 1987, in an area between Fifty-sixth and Ninety-second Streets, west of Avenue of the Americas, fifty-five studio spaces were eliminated.[90] Since small dance groups have performance seasons of a few weeks at most, performance spaces are shared. But with only a small number of these dance-performance spaces, each serving many companies, their continued existence is critical.

Because New York City is the dance capital of the world, soloists and companies need to perform there for the imprimatur of its dance critics.[91] Yet the costs are often prohibitive. When the Alwin Nikolais Company was based in New York City, it performed there infrequently. It had complicated lighting and its own technician, yet union regulations required a theater-house technician to be paid anyway.

Touring is a necessity for many dance groups to survive, since they support only a short season in most home locales. But touring, with the need to sublet one's apartment, jet lag, new foods, abrupt climatic changes, different kinds of stages, and disruption of social relationships, is stressful. Often facilities are inadequate and conducive to injury.

Some ballet companies struggling to control costs have taken up twin residencies. At one time at least ten companies had second-home arrangements. For example, the Joffrey Ballet based in New York City had a second home in Los Angeles; Cincinnati Ballet had locations in Cincinnati and New Orleans, Washington Ballet in D.C. and Baltimore, Don Wagoner and Dancers in New York and South Carolina, Cleveland Ballet in Cleveland and San Jose, Pilobolus Dance Theatre in Washington and Connecticut, Merce Cunningham in New York and Minnesota, and Pittsburgh Ballet Theatre in Pittsburgh and Savanna.

## Careers Transitions

As noted earlier, professional dancing is generally a short-term occupation. Ballet dancers tend to reach the end of their performing careers at midlife, when the body instrument begins to show decline at about thirty-five years of age. Moreover, "dance is a career dedicated to systematic downward mobility, in opposition to the general American value upon upward social mobility."[92]

> All dancers wage a losing battle against gravity and time, their bodies the instruments of betrayal in a world obsessed with youth and fairytale illusion. Airborne grace and quicksilver technique come of daunting offstage labor and a singular passion for physical perfection. With the years, the dancer's artistry gains nuance and depth, yet, paradoxically, speed, power, and flexibility begin to wane.[93]

"Tunnel vision," the refusal of dancers to acknowledge the reality of a transitory career until it is over because they are devoted solely to the physical and aesthetic demands of dancing, ultimately creates stress. Ballet dancers are not trained to think for themselves. The tip-off is stressful for older dancers: They are not cast in ballets they always danced, or they are asked to teach their roles to younger dancers. Karen Kain, a leading dancer with the National Ballet of Canada, remarked, "The very mention of retirement strikes terror in most dancers." At thirty-five, she had yet to grapple seriously with the topic personally but confessed that its inevitability haunted her. Like everyone else, she wanted to go on dancing forever but knew the day would come when she would have to be doing something else. "You're terrified that nothing will ever give you the fulfillment that dancing has given you."[94] She later became chair of the Dancer Transition Resource Centre (www.dtrc.ca), created to help dancers adjust to retirement. Other such organizations are Career Transition for Dancers (www.careertransition.org) and the International Organization for the Transition of Professional Dancers (www.iotpd.org).

Most professional ballet dancers forego college. In 1960, De Mille knew of only six choreographers of different dance forms with degrees: Birgit Cullberg, Katherine Dunham, Sybil Shearer, William Bales, Myra Kinch, and herself. Without university degrees, career transitions are often traumatic if a dancer does not choose, or have opportunities, to teach in a studio, choreograph, or work in another capacity for a dance company or arts organization. Because modern dancers commonly have a university education, it is easier for them to segue into academic dance departments. Credentials make a difference, although they are worthless in the absence of a solid track record. However, high school dropout Suzanne Farrell was able to become a tenured professor of dance at Florida State University in Tallahassee.

## Forecast

Knowledge of the trials and tribulations of a dance career certainly helps prepare an individual for its perils and alleviate some of the stress of the unknown. Yet even the older stars are often surprised by life in dance. Patrick Bissell of the American Ballet Theatre reflects:

> I thought it would be a hell of a lot more glamorous. I'm finding out you're always beat, you're always bushed. You don't have time to feel glamorous. I thought, just a few years ago, that dancing the roles I'm doing now would be a lot of fun and games, and New York would be endlessly exciting, and there would be a lot of terrific parties. Now I've found out that when there are parties, I don't go because I'm too tired.[95]

Ellen Jacob's *Dancing: A Guide for the Dancer You Can Be*[96] updated De Mille's work. A subsequent spate of autobiographies of dancers who performed with major companies reveals dimensions of the lifestyle that can sensitize the novice. In *Dance Magazine, Dancer, Dance Teacher, Dance Spirit,* and *Pointe,* you can find information about forms of dance and kinds of dance schools, criteria for evaluating these choices and your progress in the program you choose, matters of health, competitions, places to live and eat that are economically reasonable, issues of physical security in strange cities, steps toward launching a performing career, and success stories of career dancers.

Throughout the United States, clinics and hospitals provide special services for the physical and psychiatric health of dancers. There are often special days and hours and reduced rates for dancers. New knowledge, therapies, facilities, and professions have emerged to provide additional ways and sources to treat dancers. Services for dancers are frequently a division of a sports-medicine clinic.

Working in video, film, and on Broadway requires keeping up, knowing what's in, and being prepared. Market trends (in everything from dance styles to what body types are acceptable, particularly in fad-driven Los Angeles) mean dancers need to discover their professional niches within a limited window of time in order to survive fast-paced auditions and, if things go well, fast-paced jobs.

In Los Angeles, choreographer Joseph Malone tells a group he's working with:

> Shit comes really fast, right? You show up to work, they show you the stuff, and you gotta go. That's what we do, unless you get in a theatre piece; then you've got six weeks. So you have to commit whether you know what you're doing or not, like you've been doing the dance your whole frickin' life. . . . That's one of the few differences between people who work and don't work, right? There's not enough time to really rehearse it; you just gotta jump. Energy first, you'll figure the dance out second.[97]

The last decade saw hip-hop enter the market. Its mainstream popularity has hurt the livelihoods of technical jazz dancers seeking film, TV, and other commercial work. Much of the work in Los Angeles is still going to street dancers, the ones whose lives are rooted in hip-hop culture. With films like *Chicago* coming out, more technique-driven dancers are starting to work more. Now pop artists are beginning to look to technically trained dancers again—particularly that special breed who excel at the new hybrid, jazz-funk, a combination of hip-hop and jazz. Hip-hop has also brought more body types and ethnic groups on screen and in TV.

## Afterword

Given society's attitude toward dancers; the choreographer's and dance company's treatment of dancers, the hazards of injury; the low financial rewards (except for a few superstars); the economics of the dance process, production, and performance; and the brevity of a performing career, a person who pursues the dance career with all its stressors is a unique individual.

The lifestyle of a ballet dancer is similar to that of someone in a religious order, and it fulfills similar psychological needs: both religious orders and ballet institutions have a similar mortification of flesh, adoration of saints, canonization of the highly esteemed, a representation of something larger than the individual, and insistence upon giving up the self and world for a greater good. The company acts as an exterior superego driving the dancers, their individuality subdued.[98]

Passion for dance is a key motivation to pursue a dance career. Some individuals seek out dance as an occupation because of its challenges and their psychological needs; competition pushes them to greater achievements. They become accustomed to the pressures and learn how to manage the effects of stress in a constructive manner. Stress has spurred the development of new dance forms and stress-management techniques.

Mikhail Baryshnikov, ballet and movie star, says, "The stage is a form of opium for me—a psychological feeling I must have, I cannot be without."[99] Vigorous dancing induces the release of endorphins thought to produce analgesia (painlessness) and euphoria (a great high). Many professional dancers become ecstatic on a dance high that is similar to a drug-induced high but without dysphoric downer effects. This sensation generated the terms "jazzed" and "on the jazz"—and keeps dancers coming back for more. Dance teachers, such as Joe Orlando (former dance-department chairperson of the Interlochen Arts Academy) and Arthur Mitchell (artistic director of Dance Theatre of Harlem), build an infectious, euphoric spirit in the studio by exuding electric energy levels as they demonstrate for and dance with their students, some of whom get "high" and become professional dancers.

Yet some career dancers show signs of excessive stress: icy hands in a hot room; blushing, trembling extremities, shortness of breath, and furtive eyes; tears and other emotional outbursts; nervousness and increased perspiration; extra trips to the bathroom; a cry of pain due to a muscle tear. At other times a stressed dancer alone is aware of the symptoms: a palpitating heart, muscular tension, faintness, back strain, bone fracture, depression, anxiety, difficulty in swallowing, headaches, loss of appetite, intestinal and eating disorders, insomnia, a bruised psyche, feelings of frustration and resentment, and a knotted stomach. Dance teachers, students, parents, and performers alike are both victims and beneficiaries of stress.

While some dancers resort to self-destructive measures of coping with stress such as improper eating, drug abuse, and performing with injuries, others pursue dance therapy, relaxation, or counseling. Still others choose to change

careers. Efforts have been made in the dance world to alter the public perception of the performance career and to improve the working conditions of the
occupation itself to make it more like mainstream jobs with contracts, health
care, insurance, salaries, and pensions. Stress can be the spice of life or the
kiss of death.

# CHAPTER TEN

~

# Amateur Dancing in the West

Amateur dancing occurs in private and public social settings, from homes to churches, schools, and streets, to restaurants and nightclubs, and in dance classes at studios, schools, and community centers. Dance classes are offered in forms such as aerobics, African dance, ballet, ballroom, Middle East (belly dance), Brazilian dance, capoeira, classical Indian dance, flamenco, Haitian dance, hip-hop, hula, the hustle, Irish step, jazz, lyrical dance, mambo, musical comedy, salsa, samba, striptease, swing, tango, tap, and rhythm tap. Even those amateurs who do not dance in a theater for an audience, usually to show what they have learned to family and friends, are often cognizant of and affected by others watching them in social or dance-class settings.[1] Some feel self-conscious, embarrassed, or threatened because of bystanders. Thus amateur dancers may experience the kind of performance anxiety from which professional dancers suffer. Moreover, amateurs may be stressed by feelings of awkwardness and social incompetence when they fear rejection by a potential dance partner or are unable to make their feet do what the mind's eye wants them to do.

When dancers get insufficient feedback in improvisational, rather than choreographically set, social dance or in structured dance classes, to let them know whether they are doing well or poorly, they can feel stressed. In couples' social dances, a partner's response may be ambiguous. Determining whether movements are a sexual advance or merely a dance pattern is often difficult. One man explained, "You can always say you were dancing and not flirting . . . . or if you get picked up, fine."[2]

171

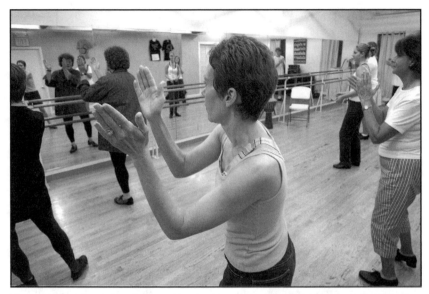

**Figure 10.1.  Tap Dance (Photo of Nancy Newell's Class at DC Dance Collective class by Dai Baker)**

Although some people attend dances out of social obligation, like weddings and other celebrations, most people choose social dances for fun. These dances tend to be a "flow activity" that helps an individual to resist and reduce stress through developing physical fitness and to escape stress through immersion in the dance. The music feeds and energizes dancers who then emanate a contagious energy that invigorates other people in the dance setting. There may be a mass elation, a *communitas,* or merging with the crowd. Dancers can communicate and interact with others, using their bodies in ways that are not done in everyday life. They can lose the self or feel in control of the self or a social situation. These dancers' comments are revealing: "Once I get into it, then I just float along, having fun, just feeling myself move around." "I get sort of a physical high from it . . . very sweaty, very feverish or sort of ecstatic when everything is going really well."[3]

Social dances often offer an opportunity for adolescents and young adults to release, with society's sanction, a variety of strong feelings that under most other circumstances they are required to suppress or repress. Each generation has its own movements, along with dress codes and music, to set itself apart, to create a sense of belonging to the "group," and to respond to its own social milieu and earlier styles. Of course, social dances permit interpersonal relations and finding sexual partners. Dancing is part of the rite of passage and courtship toward adulthood.

As is the case for professional dance, display of the instrument of dance, the body, in the amateur-dance context may enhance the dancer's self-image and thus allow her or him to resist or reduce stress. A study found, for example, that students who took folk-dance classes, when compared with those who did not take classes, were more positive about their self-concept and body image.[4]

So-called low forms of entertainment like marathons, discos, and raves have been an escape in hard economic times, much like the dances of people who confront those taking their land from them (see chapter 7). New Yorkers dealing with recession and still recovering from the 9/11 terrorist attack find refuge in the flurry of new discos that have opened in the city.

## Dance Hall Escape

In turn-of-the-20th-century New York City, working-class young women escaped from family restrictions and the tedium of work to dance halls.[5] Here they could express their sexuality in ragtime movements (the waltz, spieling, tough dancing, slow rag, lover's two-step, turkey trot, grizzly bear, and bunny hop) that would have been unacceptable in any other public forum. The dance setting was a place to go to get away from a disliked job or a conservative, nagging family. Sexuality had its stresses: Injunctions about chastity and the virtues of a woman's virginity from parents, church, and school often conflicted with the lived experience of urban labor and leisure.

> Working in factories and stores often entailed forms of sexual harassment that instructed women to exchange sexual favors for economic gain, while talk about dates and sexual exploits helped to pass the working day. Crowded tenement homes caused working-class daughters to pursue their social life in the unprotected spaces of the streets, while those living in boarding houses contended with the attentions of male lodgers. The pleasure and freedom young women craved could be found in the social world of dance halls, but these also carried a mixed message, permitting expressive female sexuality within a context of dependency and vulnerability.[6]

The dance gave the women a newfound sense of freedom at the same time the men had the prerogatives of selecting partners and breaking in on dancers. Moreover, women relied on men's treats to see them through the evening's entertainment.

## American Marathons and Argentinean Tangos

Feelings of stress due to the economy have found relief in dance. From about 1910 on, as part of a dance craze that swept the United States, social dance fads have cascaded into the popular consciousness. These dances fulfilled the same stress-relieving functions as the dances described in part II. The marathon, a special case of "besotted performance" that occurred during the Depression, coincided with changing social and cultural patterns, including heterosexual relationships.[7] The dance was called the latest form of Saint Vitus's dance, described in chapter 4.[8]

Nonstop marathons offered the dancers respite from the stress of poverty as well as catharsis and temporary escape. The marathons offered the audience empathic catharsis and divertissement from their problems. And promoters benefited financially.

Advertisements over the radio and in the papers solicited contestants. The endurance dancing of marathons attracted unemployed youth with nothing to do who were willing to suffer for the dream of a payoff, winning prize money for survival. There would usually be $1,000, a good amount at the time, which would be divided up: $600 went to the winning couple, and the last prize was $50. In addition, spectators threw money at their favorite dancers. Besides, the dancers received food and medical attention; often there was a trainer, nurse, and judge on each twelve-hour shift. George Eells, an enthusiastic audience member at countless marathons during his youth, remarked, "There was a strong personality type that was attracted to this kind of thing. I think they would've adjusted just as well to being in jail or being in the army . . . . the promoter took care of them and helped them make decisions. He got them out of jail when they were in jail; he helped them if they got into a financial bind. And then he took advantage of them and made lots of money off of them."[9] The immediacy of the marathon appealed to the audience. Every kind of person came: high school students and old ladies with their knitting; wealthy oil people who thought they were slumming; and people from the sports world, the red light district, and the middle class. The spectators could identify with the suffering the dancers projected; it made them feel better about their own problems. Some contests deteriorated into physical brutality. A former onlooker said, "I remember feeling slightly guilty about enjoying somebody else's suffering. It seemed sadistic in a way."[10] Another old-timer reflected, "People came to see 'em die. That's an overstatement. But they came to see 'em suffer, and to see when they were going to fall down. They wanted to see if their favorites were going to make it. That was all part of it. It was Depression entertainment."[11]

Some marathoners became professionals and married, divorced, and married again as they not only danced but conducted their daily tumultuous lives in public while keeping in rhythm. "It was a heightening of what you find in ordinary society because it was all enclosed in one room," said an old-timer.[12]

In the worst economic crisis in Argentina's history at the beginning of the twenty-first century, the government sponsored a nine-day tango festival in an attempt to offer some solace and diversion to the population. Dozens of free concerts, photo exhibitions, dance classes, and world competitions reaffirmed Argentine identity in a positive way. "In a crisis as terrible as this, a few hours of diversion offer a real relief from the sadness and the problems that surround us," says a dance teacher. "We've lost so much in this country. But the tango is something that is ours, that is part of our roots and cannot be taken away from us."[13]

## Rock and Disco

In the mid-1960s girls liked speeded-up dances, and boys, the unhurried ones.[14] Adolescent comments reveal dance as an escape from stress and dissipation of tension: "The more we frug, the more South Vietnam, lung cancer, and getting into your father's college fade into the distance."[15] "The dances offer temporary retreat from a complex environment with which youth seems to feel inadequately equipped to cope."[16] "The feeling is of complete thoughtlessness. The Buddhists would have called it Nirvana."[17] "It exhausts any built up strength [tension] due to anger or anxiety."[18]

Since the disco dance delirium of the 1970s, partners in many settings move as they please, independently and in unison. Revelers participate in a state of liminality, a time when social class and organizational barriers temporarily dissolve as people partake of the inverse of the bureaucratic regular world of work. The social order is rearranged on the weekend, and the week's tension is dissipated. However, living in a world in which work and dance are so bifurcated may cause stress.

## Slam Dancing

The 1980s witnessed a new dance genre in New York City and Los Angeles. Slam dancing was perhaps a way for adolescent males to deal with the stressors of maturation, aggressive personal feelings, and violence in the society at large. Through dancing, the youths expressed raw power and rage while achieving euphoria, enhanced self-concept, and a healthy fatigue.

Here is a scene from the A7 club on the Lower East Side: the crowd— 85 percent male, white, and under twenty, whether hard-core musicians, dancers or onlookers—dresses alike in "black combat boots, old Levis and black belts, almost-white T-shirts or flannel plaids, and shaved heads."[19] The

youths, mostly middle class and suburban, travel to Manhattan's tough neighborhoods to "dance dangerously and look malevolent."[20]

> The male dancers, after standing about staring at the singer, erupt on the dance
> floor.
>   Heads down, bodies hunkered over, arms flailing, they pound across the floor
> slamming into each other, the wall, and the watchers. Staggering in get-down
> fighting position, they lift up their knees, sometimes doing a spastic cross-over
> step, crashing each boot down. They slam into flesh and plaster, crash off-
> balance, and are immediately pulled up and pushed back into the tumult. They
> scramble on top of each other's shoulders, "chicken-slamming," thwacking to-
> gether, crunching to the floor in "pile-ons." Now they move into a rough circle
> "thrashing," elbows out, arms propellers, stomping and hopping like speeding
> Indians at a nightmare pow-wow. Faces grimace, eyebrows draw together.[21]

The males are ecstatic as they run amok, yet still within safety. "This activity
is about support (chicken-slams, help-ups, and push backs) and cooperation
(circle thrash). The crowd is a willing pillow. If it were really vicious, people
would simply step aside and let divers go splat. Or they could kick the shit out
of floored dancers."[22] This is not to say that there are no injuries. As with any
sport, injuries are endured as symbols of macho courage.

## Hip-Hop

The 1980s also witnessed the eruption of break dancing, the most recent
part of the former underground hip-hop social and political youth movement, with its wild-style graffiti art, special slang and clothing, and rap music. "Breaking" involves physically demanding, injury-risky, artistically inven-
tive, and pyrotechnic acrobatic and gymnastic dance movements performed
on sidewalks and in parks. These include head spins from a headstand with
hands in the air; spinning on shoulders, buttocks, or back with legs tucked
up and held by arms; freezing in pretzel forms; popping (isolating body parts
in robotlike segments so that movement ripples from one part to another);
pop-locking (fixing joints in place between movements in exaggeration for
comic effect); baby swipes (handstands in which the legs scissor sharply across
one another and the hips spiral the legs); suicides (no-hands forward flips in
which the dancer lands flat on the back); and hand glides (one hand supports the body while the other propels the body in a spin). Mime sequences
known collectively as electric boogie, for example, the wave, tick, mannequin,
walls, King Tut (imitating figures in Egyptian hieroglyphics), glides, *huevos*
(dancers walk on the toes of shoes one size larger than usual and stuffed

with newspaper), moon walks (shifting weight from one leg to the other and sliding backwards), athletic steps such as uprocking (mimed fighting and insults); toprocking (standing and performing foot movements); and shaming through mimed insults between dancers are part of the hip-hop breaking genre.

Break dancing developed in the 1970s and came to public attention from the Bronx borough of New York City. This dance form extended certain African traditions: male youth competition, innovation, self-expression, male bravura, comment on current life, and warrior dances. During the late 1960s, immigrant West African dancers and musicians began performing and teaching professional and amateur dancers in American public schools; some black Americans traveled to Africa to bring back traditions to teach and perform. Also influencing the development of break dancing were West Indian rapping (rhythmic spoken or chanted musical accompaniment), the Afro-Brazilian martial art of *capoiera*, and the African American dance repertory, including the Lindy Hop and the Charleston. The legendary James Brown's athletic, frenetic dancing to his 1969 hit song, "Get on the Good Foot," catalyzed experimentation with movement forms in which "b-boys," black and Hispanic young dancers, became proficient.

Concerned with increasing inner-city gang violence, Afrika Bambaataa, founder of the Zulu Nation, a loose confederation of Bronx dance crews, encouraged break dancing as a peaceful alternative. Intensely competitive dance "battles" occurred between warring factions. Break-dancers and onlookers would form an impromptu circle, and each performer would have a brief turn in the ring. Ghetto break-dancers expressed personal style and gained a sense of power while also conveying flamboyant, energetic group identity, values, and aesthetics. Breakdancing music was played on a recorded disco rhythm track. Common rap themes were personal self-aggrandizement and comments about women, the police, and society. Breaking was a way to be No.1 without "blowing somebody away," in some instances killing. Police arrested break-dancers, thinking they were fighting. Dancers were banned from city streets and shopping malls for causing disturbances and attracting undesirable crowds. Occasionally, a dance battle escalated into actual violence.

There are a few female break-dancers. Media obsession with break dancing popularized it nationwide. The ABC *20/20* television news program aired scenes of young street-gang members settling disputes through dance. *Mademoiselle*, *Time*, *Rolling Stone*, *People*, *Newsweek*, and the *Washington Post* have all run pieces that spotlighted break dancing. Burger King ads on television showed breaking. The first hip-hop feature film, *Wild Style*, highlighted break-dancers, as did the film *Beat Street*.

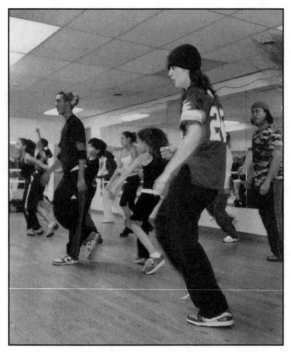

**Figure 10.2.  Hip-Hop (Photo of Rajiv Weliwitigoda's Workshop at DC Dance Collective by Judith Lynne Hanna)**

Outstanding break-dancers gained financial rewards by performing on the street, in theaters, at birthday parties and bar mitzvahs, through club bookings and international tours, and on television and film. They gave hip-hop classes without the break-dance pyrotechnics at college campuses, grade schools, dance studios, gyms, and sports and recreation centers.

Break dancing soon crossed racial and ethnic boundaries and spread among young people in America and abroad. The media hype eventually altered break dancing's form and meaning. The circular format became linear; the style became standardized with less improvisation, acrobatics, and "freeze" (a held, often seemingly impossible, position of personal and group expression). Like many popular dances, break dancing became part of the formalized history of black folklore, but by the 1980s, street kids felt breaking no longer belonged to them and went on to create new dances. The easier-to-do moves like poppin' and lockin' entered hip-hop classes for all ages and sexes that were taught by studio-dance teachers.

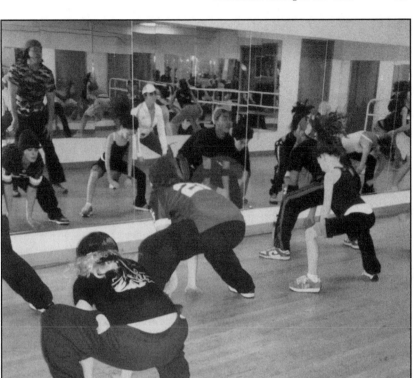

Figure 10.3.   Hip-Hop (Photo of Rajiv Weliwitigoda's Workshop at DC Dance Collective class by Judith Lynne Hanna)

## Raves

Held in different places, rave dances (also called clubbing) originated in the 1980s in Europe and developed in the 1990s in the United States as part of an underground culture.[23] Concerts around the country were broadcast on the raveworld.net Web site. Rave sponsors usually rent a warehouse on the pretext of doing a video, ten to fifteen DJs provide techno-house and hip-hop music, and about three to four thousand people in their early teens to early twenties attend throughout the night. The DJs are like shamans in cultures that have odd hours for unusual ritual activities. Raves have been associated with drugs, especially the euphoria-inducing ecstasy, which reduces people's self-con-sciousness and fear of censure so they can lose themselves in the joy of dancing.

Dancers seek to experience altered states of consciousness and a transcen-dental spiritual affirmation of life through dancing en masse all night to a throbbing repetitive music beat and hypnotic light show. A common reason to attend raves appears to be to express one's youthful identity as different from and contrary to mainstream society and one's parents' generation. Find-ing themselves in a world they did not make or approve of, rave dancers cut the umbilical cord. Moreover, reflecting sexual equality, young women go by them-selves and dance without male partners.

Like the dance halls and marathons of the past, raves are a form of escape from a world in turmoil with pressures to succeed. Raves provide release in a secure and safe environment and a vehicle to communicate emotion, a subjec-tively experienced state of feeling. Dancing in communal settings often builds up infectious joy and identification with or inclusion in a culture or group, which prevent or reduce emotions such as alienation. "Dancing . . . unleashes the Dionysian body from the Apollonian constraints imposed on it in the everyday world," says anthropologist Phil Jackson about the clubbing scene in England.[24] A male informant told him, "If you haven't fucked God on a dance floor, then you've never truly danced."[25] Many rave dancers follow the mantra of PLUR: Peace, love, unity, and respect. The dancing evolved from hip-hop and includes popping and locking and running man (running in place). Raves may reduce stress or allow the dancer to develop physical fitness to resist stress.

## Carnival

Throughout the Western world, Carnival (aka Mardi Gras) occurs before the Lenten period (a Christian symbolic penitence from Ash Wednesday to Easter). The festival originated in the second century in Rome when the fast of the forty days of Lent was preceded by a feast lasting several days during which time participants put on masks and costumes and considered all pleasure allowable. The modern world's carnival is likened to the Saturnalia of the Christian Romans. That spread to other European countries and finally to the Americas and the Caribbean. Carnival has been observed in the United States, most notably, in New Orleans from 1827 when a group of students, recently returned from school in Paris, donned strange costumes, and danced their way through the streets trying to replicate the revelry they had experienced in Paris. Today immigrants from the Caribbean and South America hold their own unrestrained celebrations with energetic dancing to the seething samba, salsa, and reggae beats.

Brazil is renowned for its samba schools, street festivities, competitions, and elegant masquerade balls. Carnival in Rio has been called the world's most famous party. A million tourists join millions of Rio de Janeiro citizens (*cariocas*) in enthusiastic revelry spanning several days. The highlight is the half-mile-long Sambodromo parade of the fourteen best samba schools, flanked by spectator stands and luxury boxes. There are also street processions of other samba schools. Sounds and sights of the parading samba schools go on from dusk to daybreak.

A samba school is typically a group from a poor neighborhood organized to produce a lavish Carnival procession for fun. Each samba school has showy floats with sensuous women vibrating to hypnotic music. Marching samba bands numbering up to three hundred musicians surrounded by a sea of flamboyantly or scantily clad singer/dancers accompany the floats. These diverse parade elements work as a single unit, dramatizing the same theme, which the samba school changes annually. A school can have up to four thousand participants. Carnival preparation requires nearly a year of sewing, building, composing, choreographing, and rehearsing. Taking a sizable slice of their income, samba school participants pay for their own extravagant costumes adorned with feathers, lamé, masks, and papier-mâché heads. They willingly do this because Carnival is a fantasy escape from their hardscrabble lives. Major samba schools in Rio spend up to $300,000 per year preparing for Carnival.

Masquerade balls for the elite are celebrity-attended affairs. The merrymakers wear designer costumes and party from before midnight to the wee hours. The ball at the Copacabana Palace Hotel is the most famous.

## Swing Revivals

Foreigners have been fueling a revival of one of America's hottest dance crazes, popular dances from the 1920s to the 1950s. Dancers today view old films of the original Lindy Hoppers. Some of these old-timers share knowledge of the best material danced on the Savoy Ballroom floor in Harlem.[26] And teachers disseminate how to swing, which includes dances called the Lindy Hop, Fall off the Log, Charleston, Sugar Push, Balling the Jack, Trucking, Susie Q, the Big Apple, and Shim Sham, at dance studios, community centers, workshops, and dance camps. Many people enjoy the spontaneous and uninhibited spirit, impeccable timing, partner call and response, smooth grounding, and high energy. The advanced and daring dancer performs over-the-shoulder aerials with acrobatic skill and impressive dips (in which the lead lowers his partner close to the ground).

## Folk Dancing

Amateur folk dancing allows people to cope with stress in a variety of ways, including escaping from technological society and returning to human contact. One dancer explains: "Folk dancing keeps things on a human plane . . . . Part of the etiquette of contra dancing is the eye contact." Another says, "It's great for business travel. You get to a new town, call someone from the folk dance network and spend the evening dancing. There's no other social activity in which you touch someone the same evening you meet them." Yet another man agrees: "Where else can you spend $4 and put your hands on a hundred women?"[27]

## The Ballroom Dance Studio

An upcoming wedding catapults many a bride and groom, their parents, and members of the wedding party to learn ballroom dances (ballroom dancing is also a professional career). Adults generally seek skills utilized in the "polite companionship" of social dancing.[28] Ballroom studios also attract another group: defenseless and lonely people who want relations with the opposite sex—affection, trust, reciprocity, and concern with mutual feelings—so badly that they are willing to use studios to buy them. The studio puts on regular or special event "parties" that duplicate social occasions on the outside. Students, teachers, and teacher trainees are encouraged to bring guests to the studio to witness lessons or attend the parties, for guests are an important source of new students.

In addition to the potential stress amateurs experience, students get upset when the ballroom dance studio activities are the means to neither develop the social skills of moving, talking, and dressing nor acquire social relationships with the teachers and other students after substantial monetary expenditures. Upon discovering the actual cost for the services, students are often shocked. In the early 1970s there were exposés by information media, lawsuits by allegedly victimized persons, and negative side smiles by society at large.[29] Over thirty years ago, "lessons at chain schools cost between $5 and $9 per half-hour or $10 to $18 for the standard one hour. Studios attempted to enroll students for at least 100 hours but, as several well-publicized lawsuits have pointed out, women have been known to sign up for lessons totaling more than $10,000."[30] Management pressures the teachers not only to teach the students to dance but also to sign them up for "renewals" for large blocks of lessons or even for lifetime courses.

## A Ballet Class

Physical fitness and escape from everyday stresses are the bounty of the dance class for some students. Linda Valleroy observes herself and other ballet hobbyists:

> Up the stairs in your business clothes. You hear the piano playing Chopin. You are beat, but suddenly begin to feel a little happier. Into the practice clothes, the shoes. You talk to some girlfriends about how the Kirov is coming to town. Already you are feeling a lot happier and then class starts. Concentrate. Keep the flow of energy moving. Don't sit in the plies. Pull up the knees. Oops, there goes that stupid tension in my arm, again. How can I ever keep my pelvis parallel in *rond de jambes*? God, they are hard. They have always been hard. This is the litany of the anatomy.
>
> Now, after all these years of ballet I am starting on a new system. I play anatomy class at the barre and really try to dance in the center. Sometimes I really dance. But you know, it's a few seconds here, a few seconds there. Anyway, by the end of class I am generally always so happy. The others are happy, too. You just have to close your eyes and listen to the voice quality in the dressing room. People talk faster. Their voices are high pitched. And, I keep wondering what did it. What was it that made the world seem like an enchanting place, again? Whatever it was is what keeps me paying my seven dollars there as opposed to some wine bar.[31]

Valleroy reflects upon what seems to create the euphoria: Because one focuses on a complicated set of anatomical maneuvers, all the body placement positions, the flow of energy, the quality of the movement, and tempo of the music, there is no time to think about one's identity and problems. The individual mentally and physically realigns the body, because ballet is a unique postural system that requires an uplifting posture. Mastery over the body and greater physical fitness leads to self-confidence. So does enlarging one's social network. Class is planned continuous movement that lasts an hour or more, and endorphin levels are highest in exercise over an hour. Valleroy thinks the ballet dance class is a

> regression to a childhood state, far, far, from the adult professional world. Many women in adult ballet classes are career women who struggle with adult [and feminine] problems in a man's world during the [playless work] day. At night you can be a little kid again, or a swan, or a princess. These mental images will not get one very far in the work world. What a relief to be a swan.

## Aerobic Dance and Jazzercise

Aerobic dance has the potential for physical and psychological benefits. This genre combines simple dance patterns. Evidence of psychological benefits comes from a study of female teachers who participated in an aerobic-dance program in an educational employment setting. The teachers showed decreased symptoms of burnout and improved relations with their colleagues as well as with administrators. Moreover, the teachers' students found their teachers to be more knowledgeable, poised, lively, and interesting.[32] Jazzercise combines jazz dance like aerobic and strength-training exercises. The franchise is national and individuals can go to a class anywhere and know the routines.

## Afterword

Individuals participate in social dancing or dance classes for pleasure, exercise, a way of marking self-identity, and meeting and interacting with other people. The dance may help individuals to resist stress through developing physical fitness and building social support that extends beyond the dance setting. Reduction of stress may occur through the dissipation of quotidian tensions of work and family as well as crises such as economic depression or war. Escape from stress occurs through the flow and ecstasy of multisensory envelopment or the fantasy and enchantment of a romantic dance genre. Amateur dance may induce stress through performance anxiety, insufficient social-dance invitations, inadequate dance-class support from teacher or classmates, and ambiguous performance feedback.

~

## CHAPTER ELEVEN

# Dance/Movement Therapy

## Body Language: Theoretical Underpinnings

Dance/movement therapy (DMT) is the Western psychotherapeutic use of movement, which emerged in the 1940s. DMT is a process that helps a person get it all together, that is, it furthers the physical, emotional, and cognitive integration of an individual. Some therapists prefer the term "dance" to "movement" because the former is associated with joy and well-being. Moreover DMT certification requires many years of dance training. The American Dance Therapy Association, formed in 1966, has its own journal and list of certified therapists. DMT has spread to more than thirty-one countries, some of which have their own associations and publications.[1] In addition to therapists who are certified in DMT, psychologists, psychiatrists, counselors, social workers, and sensitivity trainers may use dance or movement in therapy. Many practitioners consider specific ritual dances, such as the ones that have been described in earlier chapters, to be the genesis of the therapeutic use of dance in the West. Others claim modern dance is the source.

Because DMT is relatively new and has diverse practices, I will return to some aspects of the theory in part I and comment on specific DMT models. DMT's theoretical approaches help to explain how and why DMT differs from other forms of dance. Note that the term "stress" is not as common in the literature of DMT as other concepts that can be subsumed under stress, such as anxiety, insecurity, isolation, and alienation. The latter part of the chapter will present some cases DM therapists have described.

Nonverbal communication, the bodily sending and receiving of messages, is integral to the dance/movement healing process and makes it unique among Western forms of therapy. The expressive body movement is assumed to reveal aspects of a person's state of mind, personality, emotions, feelings, and range of adaptive behaviors. Therapists recognize that movement communication may support or contradict verbal behavior, and, furthermore, that people may be able to communicate better through nonverbal than verbal means. So, too, therapists hold the premise that individual growth and well-being depend on self-expression. Practitioners believe that because mind and body interact, a change in a client's movement expression affects the person's total functioning and allows experimentation with new ways of being.[2] A person may have the sensation of both moving and being moved.

A DM therapist assists a person to work through problems in order to gain insight, change behavior, establish emotional contact with other humans, and release tension. DM therapists observe an individual's or family's movements for diagnostic purposes, treatment goals, and assessment of change over time as a result of therapy.[3] Practitioners read a client's posture, gesture, face, use of space (distance between her- or himself and others), synchrony with others, manner of touch, and eye gaze. Training in dancer Rudolf Laban's methods (as developed by his disciples) of analyzing and symbolically representing dynamic and spatial aspects of movement helps in observing and recording movement during a therapy session. For example, scientific research seeks movement parameters that indicate suicidal risk and other less-severe stress responses.

DMT may be an integral component of a broad treatment program or a primary intervention. The condition of a client in DMT varies; a client may be under acute or chronic traumatic stress or may be experiencing minor stress. Therapists may treat severely disturbed patients in psychiatric hospitals and other long-term institutions, and other clients in community health centers, nursing homes, private practice offices, clinics, special educational settings, and the therapist's or client's home. DM therapists may work with staff in a mental-health setting to sensitize the staff to their own movement behavior and the movement of patients so that staff behavior becomes more effective in interaction with patients.

The pattern of interpersonal relations varies in DMT sessions. Therapy may take place solely in a dyadic therapist-client interaction, with a client's family, or in a group that includes the therapist and several or more clients. Interpersonal dancing is designed to enhance empathy and trust between individuals. A group dancing together is potentially nurturing for some clients.

Among its many uses, dance/movement therapy aims to help people overcome trauma, often by nonverbally bringing the elements of the experience to the fore. A retelling, a giving testimony, can help to make sense of the incomprehensible and transform the surreal into something real. Under the protective cloak of therapy, clients who suffer bewilderment, dislocation, and revisited negative emotions from traumatic stress can access their own personality resources to help them to transform these feelings.[4] For those who have suffered first-hand trauma and second-hand witnessing of images on television, video, or the Internet, DMT may follow the approach of Chris Brewin, an internationally recognized expert on trauma (see chapter 1).[5] Treatment involves the need to expose a client to traumatic information and modify maladaptive beliefs about events, behavior, or symptoms. The cues to retrieving memories need to be associated with a sense of current safety. Violently inflicted pain on the body usually requires a restoration of the sense of accepting the "dirtied" body, integration of the separated body and soul, and rebuilding social relationships.[6]

DMT does not use a standard dance form or movement technique. Any genre, from African folk to European waltz, may be drawn upon. Improvisation is common. Much of what is called dance therapy does not appear to be what we usually call dance but is rather movement or types of dance warm-up exercises. A therapist may mirror a client's muscle-tension changes and body shape in a show of empathy. Some therapists use somatic body therapies (see below), Dalcroze rhythmic methods, yoga's striving for inner peace, and Dervish turning to achieve altered states of consciousness. Many therapists attempt to have clients alleviate tension to facilitate the flow of expression by making use of the full range of movement qualities that have been described by Laban and his followers.[7] Issues of dependency, fight-flight, and pairing come to the fore.

The reason for such variety in DMT lies in the therapist's background and training in addition to the broad spectrum of populations that undergo DMT. There are self-actualizers (individuals who cope well with daily life but desire to be more in touch with their expressive body actions), neurotics, psychotics, the mentally retarded, individuals suffering from sociopathic conditions (delinquents, battered women, drug addicts), individuals who are physically challenged, and the elderly.

## Theoretical Underpinnings

The underpinning for DMT comes from the human potential, holistic health approaches, or medical models. The humanistic and holistic health approaches have in common the belief that individuals share responsibility for their therapeutic progress and relationships with others. By contrast, the medical model assumes that the therapist is primarily responsible for treatment and cure.

There are various, but not usually mutually exclusive, theoretical approaches to dance therapy that do not necessarily require different physical techniques.[8] DMT is grounded in the worlds of dance and psychology. Some DMT approaches, such as Marian Chace's pioneering work,[9] derive from experimentation with dance; other approaches derive from psychoanalysis or are aligned with behavior modification. The majority of therapists ascribe to one or more theoretical frames of reference such as the following:

Psychoanalysis, developed by Sigmund Freud, offers DMT a diagnostic tool in its theory of stages of physical and psychological maturation. The Freudian developmental theory assumes that through therapy the client outgrows an inefficient, fixated, or infantile mode and dissolves resistance to maturation. A vital concept is transference: people become emotionally engaged with the therapist as a stand-in for a significant figure out of the past. In therapy, the psychological moment in a person's life when she or he suffered hurts may be re-created so that the person may see how this was experienced and thus gain insights for an improved life. The individual's psychological makeup, conflicts, and defenses manifest themselves in the dance process, which is seen as a symbolic reflection of the psychological state of the individual and a vehicle to a new state of mind. Freud emphasized the body as the basis of the ego, the part of the self that mediates between inner strivings and outer demands. Motility is, therefore, part of the ego apparatus. DMT helps to release and sublimate repressed psychosexual and aggressive impulses.

Within the psychoanalytic field, the work of Wilhelm Reich, C. Gustav Jung, and Henry Stack Sullivan, among others, guides DMT. Reich was concerned not only with what a patient said, but how the person moved. He believed that the individual's walk, stance, and breath patterns revealed a specific character type. Reich thought chronic muscular tension indicated repression and blocked the expression of affect. An example is the tight holding of the chest area as a sign of repressed feelings of need and longing. DMT attempts to reduce muscular tension, what Reich calls the "defensive armor," to facilitate regained mobility.

Within the Jungian approach, dance is viewed as an expression of healing rather than a projection of personality or psychopathology and evidence of disease and disorder. Art is considered the means by which patients may objectify themselves. Participation in DMT evokes conscious and unconscious fantasies and conflicts, that are then available for analysis and catharsis.

Sullivan's interpersonal theory of personality contends that the individual develops through the accumulated experience of self in interaction with others. The experience or perception of the interaction, rather than its objectivity, is what matters in this process. Therapists following Sullivan attempt to resocialize the individual's interpersonal style with other people in order to develop more-successful nonstressful social relationships.

Learning theory considers dance as a basic need and a safe insulated arena through which to explore feelings and thoughts in order to renew old values or introduce new ones and thereby change behavior. The orientation of communication theory is that different ways of expression and communication may be blocked, congruent, or conflicting. Mediated by dance, insights facilitate verbal reflexivity and resolution of conflicting messages. The cognitive-behavior approach seeks through dance to reverse faulty thinking patterns and negative feelings about the self.

Gestalt-phenomenological theory emphasizes awareness, excitement, and involvement (responsibility and contact) in the moment-to-moment process of living,[10] This approach precludes the therapist's predetermined judgment and movement structure. Instead, by spontaneously responding to a new situation, a DM therapist helps someone acquire self-knowledge and acceptance in order to grow.

Psychomotor-developmental theory posits that individuals who have difficulty adapting can improve their lives by recouping those movement components that they did not experience in the normal growth process. The pragmatic approach assumes that a DM therapist should be able to deal with any kind of situation, since other modes of therapy may be unavailable. Practitioners of this orientation draw upon whatever theory and method seems most applicable to the client's condition.

An Australian dance therapy developed to accommodate the range of ethnic groups, practitioner backgrounds, and demographic settings in that country; it departs from theoretical constructions that place dance therapy exclusively in the realm of psychotherapy. Rather the focus is humans dancing further into health. An aesthetic component is essential. The five-phase journey begins with entry, the process of the client's acceptance of dance as a therapeutic medium. Trust through the therapist's unconditional positive regard for the client and empathic responses are critical. However, therapists also need to be concerned with personal safety; a client may arrive in an aroused state, be anxious, and strike out. Second, exploration, through guided movement or improvisation, helps the therapist to discover what led to the client's current condition. Spontaneous movements begin to express intrapsychic aspects of the client, and movement becomes metaphoric. Selected movements from themes are developed and clarified in the third stage, core action. Insights emerge. In the fourth phase, review, the dance experience is grounded in the real world and its relevance to daily living is reflected on. Conclusion is the cessation of therapy when clients feel confident of managing their lives more productively.[11]

On the basis of group-therapy theory and clinical experience, Claire Schmais offers a preliminary categorization of eight interrelated healing processes in guided group DMT.[12] These processes operate in many of the ritual, social, and theatrical dances mentioned earlier that help people to resist, reduce, and escape stress: (1) Synchrony refers to people moving together in time or making the same spatial design with the same body parts, or effort, irrespective of body parts. Movement synchrony is often supported by touch, visual contact, and/or sounds and words toward promotion of group solidarity, resocialization, and expression. (2) Expression as a goal is predicated on the notion that externalization of internal states makes them less ominous, especially in a group setting that provides a supportive matrix for shameful and frightening feelings. (3) Rhythm serves to integrate, inspire, and regulate the DMT participation process. (4) Vitalization, investing people with the power to live, occurs through moving. "The flow of motion connects limbs to torso and feelings to actions.... In the dance therapy session there is a synergistic effect resulting from the stimulation of being in a group situation and from the activation that is caused by moving."[13] (5) Integration in DMT describes the dynamic accomplishment of a sense of unity within the individual and a sense of community between internal and external reality. Schmais explains:

> For most patients, the accretive process begins with a simple motion, perhaps a flick of the wrist. The therapist repeats the movement, adding descriptive phrases and poetic images to enhance the meaning and crystallize the action. As the energy level rises, the gesture of a single joint can become a postural motion spreading through the entire body, cutting through tension and engaging inert areas. The facial expressions, sounds, and words become congruent with the body actions. Body parts connect, discordant rhythms disappear, and distracting gestures dissolve.[14]

(6) Cohesion refers to the social bond that exists in dance content and form. Steps toward people actively participating in each other's symbolic statements include the group connecting through the rhythmic beat, auditory and visual feedback from members of the group, physical closeness, and touching, first of oneself to experience self-awareness and then of others such as in a light tapping of another's shoulder or hand. When the group dances out a person's

private story, the storyteller finds group and self-acceptance.[15] (7) Education refers to clients learning from their own experiences as well as from others, especially through participating in their symbolic expressions. For example, a patient mirroring another person's dancing out a theme of sorrow may express her or his own unfinished mourning and gain awareness of how other people deal with loss and the necessity of accepting the inevitability of death. "As the group affect escalates, patients see others change and realize that they too are changing, and that change is possible. . . . Coming to the sessions with anxiety, annoyance, and little enthusiasm, patients learn that the act of moving itself can reduce tensions, diminish depression, and increase energy. . . . By being trusted to support someone else or to lead the group, they learn to trust themselves and to take initiative. And when powerful feelings are exposed as part of the dance, patients learn that expressing emotions does not necessarily lead to disaster."[16] (8) Symbolism is "probably the least understood and most valuable process in dance therapy. It requires a certain technical mastery to abstract and structure what is seen, felt, and imagined. . . . Symbolic expressions in dance therapy form the bridge between the patient's internal and external worlds as they transfer energy from one realm to the other in a social context" to allow for psychic distance from private preoccupations.[17] See the finale for discussion on finding meaning in movement.

Neuropsychiatrist David Akstein[18] capitalized on his understanding of possession states (discussed in chapters 3–5) to develop a new type of group psychotherapy called Terpsichoreotrance therapy (TTT). Following the practice of trance in Brazilian religious sects, TTT trance is supported by music from the Umbanda sect and is performed in a theatrical setting. TTT, however, discards the mystic. Members of the social class to which the patient is accustomed comprise the therapy group. TTT technique bears some resemblance to hypnosis. Although a director gives instructions for clients to close their eyes and concentrate on one thing they wish to accomplish to increase their rate of breathing (hyperventilation), no other oral communication with clients occurs. Every client has an assistant on the alert nearby so that falls do not occur. Clients may dance the samba, sway, or burst into violent trance. Those who develop a deep trance dance slowly, display a tranquil countenance, and achieve a sense of well-being after the session. The calmness gives the patient the means to better face and solve problems.

Therapy based on Eastern Buddist philosophy, such as the human-potential model at the Naropa Institute (discussed in chapter 9) aims to awaken and to uplift people. The artistic process is seen as part of everyday life and that everyone is an artist.[19]

## Cultural Sensibilities

Since the body is composed of universal features, some members of the Western medical and therapeutic professions who use DMT erroneously assume that the body is experienced in a universal manner,[20] including how it uses the elements of dance, namely, time, space, and energy. When cultural norms are violated in the DMT process, stress is induced rather than alleviated. Norine Dresser offers some guidance for general interpersonal behavior in her book, *Multicultural Manners: New Rules of Etiquette for a Changing Society.*[21]

However, therapists today generally recognize that cultural learning plays a role in the biological and psychic behavior of humans and that cultures themselves are not homogeneous. Cultures have internal variations based on age, gender, ethnicity, race, religion, language, occupational group, immigration period (first or second generation), and so on. The physically challenged, mentally disturbed, and mentally retarded may be conceived of as having their own cultures. Cross-cultural and social-class problems are particularly evident in urban areas, where most publicly and privately supported professional dance training and therapy occur. Given cultural and intracultural variation, the specific movement patterns of emotions may also vary (see chapter 2).

Over the years, America has welcomed refugees from many troubled places in the world—Europe, Latin America, and Asia. Vietnam, Cambodia, Somalia, Ethiopia, El Salvador, Nepal, Pakistan, to name but a few countries, are represented in the United States. Involuntary minorities, groups that did not choose to become part of the United States but were forced against their will, include American Indians, Alaskan natives, Mexicans living in the Southwest prior to its conquest, native Hawaiians, Puerto Ricans, and blacks brought to the United States as slaves. The ways these groups have interpreted and responded to their situations of mistreatment by white Americans affect their attitude to white institutions and practices. Their individual and community experiences with discrimination have led some to distrust white institutions and practices and to exhibit defensive oppositional behavior.

Because humans spin webs of significance from their own cultural perspectives, therapists are most successful when they understand how individual clients, as well as the cultures to which they belong, view the cause of a problem and the progress of its resolution. Movements, usually possessing little meaning in and of themselves, reveal meaning only within the larger pattern of behavior of which they are a part. The body has many components, each of which may send a different message. Consequently, knowing the context of how individuals learn to move and how appropriate the movement is according to their groups is critical.

So, too, is knowing the cultural conceptions of educational and therapeutic approaches—the criteria for who participates in dance, when, where, and how; and what movements are preferred, prescribed, and proscribed. This knowledge can determine, for example, whether it would be preferable to opt for creative or imitative techniques and to select individual or group interaction. Resisting and reducing stress in many societies involves a mobilization of personal networks. Consequently, effective therapy may require the participation of persons who radiate outward from the stressed person (family, friends, and neighbors).

## Illustrative Cases

### Therapists' Therapy

Therapists themselves seek dance therapy from other therapists in order to deal with the stresses they encounter in their work. Supervision and peer support from people who are aware of the problems are sources of help for the therapist in resisting and reducing the stresses of trying to help clients.

The stressful treatment situation with schizophrenic patients may lead the therapist to react with defensive or compensatory responses.[22] These reactions may help the therapist sustain an investment in the patient and a commitment to the treatment process at the same time that the responses may be counterproductive to the patient's treatment. Susan Sandel's work at Yale Psychiatric Institute and her supervision of practicing DM therapists reveals four interrelated issues. First, the therapist's perceived hopelessness of a treatment situation often leads to the therapist's omnipotent fantasies. This defensive reaction may protect the therapist from feeling despair. However, it may also lead the therapist to perceive improvement in a patient that other clinicians do not see. Second, the intensity of the therapist's emotional involvement with the patient may make the therapist feel the threat of being overwhelmed. Third, a schizophrenic's lack of responsiveness challenges the therapist's ability. Fourth, the therapist is vulnerable to the effects of the schizophrenic's sensitivity to her or his unconscious processes. "The therapist's struggle to protect and develop his or her investment in the patient while remaining open to experiencing the hopelessness, anger, and even disorganization stimulated by his or her contact with the patient, emerges in a particular way for the dance therapist. It is affected by both the historical development of dance therapy and the nature of the movement experience."[23] Sandel recalls an experience of feeling adequate and the need for therapy herself. She had worked hard during a group therapy session in which all the patients were involved, expressing feelings and creating images. At the end of the session, thinking she was doing a fine job, she asked the group with anticipation how people felt about the session. There was silence. She looked about expectantly, "and one patient said innocently, 'What session?' "[24]

Therapists who try to help victims of incest tend to feel stress. In supervising therapists, Judith Bunny structures movement exercises to help the therapists meet the pressures of working through the incest victim's family dynamics and emotions. Caring for the Caregiver is the signature program of workshops and performance work designed by Stuart Pimsler Dance and Theater (SPDT) to help health-care professionals find expression for the complex emotional issues and unacknowledged stress associated with their work. Since introducing the program in 1992 at Shands Hospital in Gainesville, Florida, SPDT has worked with a broad cross section of the health-care community (physicians, nurses, medical students, hospice staff and volunteers, social workers, therapists, counselors, administrative personnel, and patients and their families). Each workshop is tailored to a group's particular needs. Commonly, following a movement warm-up, a series of improvisational exercises allows each participant to move and verbalize at her or his own level of skill and comfort. For example, focusing on issues of support, participants share personal stories and reflections on how they provide support in their daily work. Then with a partner, participants explore the physical realm of support. They take turns experiencing holding and being held, supporting and being supported, trusting and being trusted. Discussion follows. In a workshop titled "Out of This World," participants bring their life-and-death experiences to the stage to move through them and pose such universal questions as, What's it like to die? What's the value of saying good-bye? They explore how loss resonates in the body and in memory.

What happens when a dance therapist is physically incapacitated? Dancer and dance therapist Marcia Plevin offers one answer.[25] Having begun the Martha Graham technique at eleven years of age, trying to please her instructors, she thinks she overdid it. At sixteen she demonstrated for the technique classes. After being a dance major at the University of Wisconsin, she danced in New York City with members of the Martha Graham Company and began doing her own choreography. At thirty, she was on the modern-dance faculty of the North Carolina School of the Arts. "My hips began to give me trouble when I was around 35."[26] Her hips caused much pain, constricting rotation, jiggles, and sways. Walking, sitting, and making love were difficult. She had a left-hip replacement, which ended up causing her left hip to be higher than the right hip. Six weeks later she returned to teaching modern-dance technique at the National Italian Academy for Dance, seeing clients, and walking slowly with a lift in her shoe. Ten months later she had the right hip replaced, but by a different surgeon.

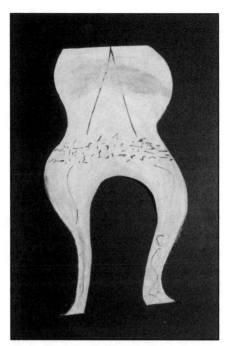

Figure 11.1.  Dancing Colors (by Marcia Plevin, dancer/artist/dance movement therapist)

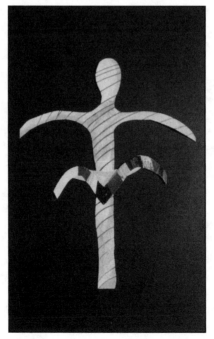

Figure 11.2.  Dancing Colors (by Marcia Plevin, dancer/artist/dance movement therapist)

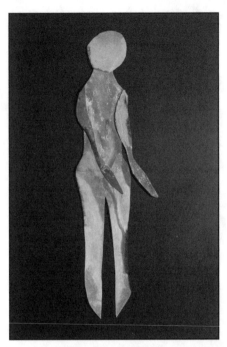

Figure 11.3. Dancing Colors (by Marcia Plevin, dancer/artist/dance movement therapist)

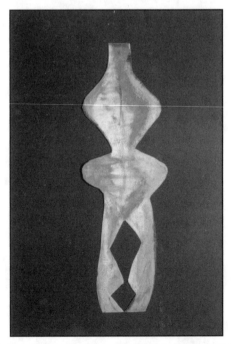

Figure 11.4. Dancing Colors (by Marcia Plevin, dancer/artist/dance movement therapist)

Unable to move, and needing to help her movement healing process, Plevin discovered "color dancing," which brought her gracefully through the recovery period from two hip prosthetic operations. Plevin explains color dancing: "Throughout the two operations I became a creative arts therapist for myself. The creative process, the basis of dance therapy, was channeled into writing and creating art and poetry.... Creativity came through parts of the body that could respond... [it has been] a true godsend." In her sixth decade of life, she is feeling great.

## Women's Issues
In a women's dance-movement therapy group, members dance out imagery focused on death and violence, including forced abortion and molestation. As the body has been invaded, all normal physical and emotional boundaries have been disregarded. Sexual violation is often experienced as a trauma to every aspect of the being. Moreover, violation by family members, religious leaders, and teachers is a breach of love and trust. When women make profound links between these disclosed events and their own feelings of revulsion at certain parts of their bodies, the therapist leads the group in dancing to reclaim those body parts.

Survivors live with emotional scars, among them injured self-concept, guilt, shame, depression, relationship problems, and sexual dysfunction. Women talk about how they inhibit themselves in their lives out of guilt and lack of self-trust. Dealing with survivors of traumatic sexual abuse, therapist Bonnie Bernstein leads groups to "let go" physically.[27] She begins a therapy session with a directive to explore a range of arm and leg movements in a variety of directions in space to discover "stepping out in new ways" on different levels. Using movement as a bridge to coping with stress-laden themes, she asks each group member to describe how she might be stepping out in new ways in her life. A victim spoke of letting a neighbor into her home, which was a new behavior because she usually kept everyone out. This habit reflected the shame and secrecy that surrounded the home where the trauma occurred. A rape survivor moved at a slow tempo that inhibited joyous excitement, muted sexual passion, and demonstrated an inability to express anger. In sessions where she experimented with varying her tempo, using photographs from her youth to capture energy, she realized her fear of her rapist's rageful violence had robbed her of free expression.

One group enacted the story of Harriet Tubman, the woman who escaped both slavery and an abusive husband and went on to be a legendary conductor of the Underground Railroad. The women integrated aspects of the Tubman story with their own tragic situations.

A therapist can help a client confront her unrealistic psychophysical distortions as they emerge in dance/movement expression.[28] For example, a therapist suggested an image of "reaching for what you want," to which the client responded by reaching toward an open window moving her arms as if to fly away and then desisted, perceiving the impossibility of escape from her boyfriend. The therapist asked her to consider realistic options for avoiding her abuser. She then realized she could begin to distance herself by altering her work schedule and thus begin to plan the next move.

With some training concerning domestic violence and working alongside a social worker, Gina Gibney heads an all-female six-member company that offers an outreach program to help survivors of domestic abuse reclaim their lives and bodies through dance. Gibney works in shelters operated by Safe Horizons in New York City. In contrast to what the women have been told (that they are dumb and ugly) and how they have been controlled within confined strictures, the dance class is a safe place in which the women have choices and can improve their self-concept.[29]

Female victimization may be perpetuated to the point of causing psychological paralysis such that pervasive apprehension and terror lead to a victim's cutting off feeling, detaching and dissociating herself from experience she feels she cannot control; she may assign her feelings to the abuser who batters her. Dance therapy works toward having the victim embody independent actions and experience conscious choice. Directed creative movement addresses patterns of isolation, helplessness, ambivalence, and immobilization. Broadening movement patterns symbolically increase the range of action and interaction—change often occurs in movement before it occurs elsewhere. Dance can help rebuild physical and emotional sensations a victim previously disowned to allow her to become whole again.

### Migration

Americans migrating to rural areas in order to escape the stresses of city living may find adjusting to the different environment difficult. They often feel alienation from established residents, the isolation of country living, the lack of jobs, and winter cabin fever. Dance is among the useful therapeutic coping techniques.[30] Of course, going to the big city from rural areas or small towns can be overwhelming. Immigrants without legal entry documentation face a host of problems.

### Aging

There is no question that aging brings new stress to one's life. The increasing American population of seniors faces diminished physical well-being, loneliness, insecurity, depression, confusion, anxiety, and anger. The U.S. Bureau of the Census reported that the number of sixty year olds has doubled to 43 million over the last two decades and is likely to reach 83 million by 2030. Because seniors often suffer the stress of physical and mental deterioration resulting from the aging process, neurological diseases or injuries, ways to ameliorate the stresses are crucial. Dancing ameliorates some effects of aging—decline in mental functioning and discomfort through building fitness and endurance.[31] Dance therapy has the ability to improve dynamic balance, rhythmic discrimination, and memory. This therapy has fostered personal interaction, self-initiated activities, and decision making. In studies, seniors have found DMT pleasurable and reported enhanced mood, energy, social relations, energy, and physical well-being. Liz Lerman addresses the benefits and approaches to dance for senior citizens.[32]

Sandel worked among nursing-home residents, and longing for companionship, fear of physical deterioration, and sexual frustration commonly emerged in their movement-therapy sessions. She found that sound and movement activities create an atmosphere of excitement that revitalize geriatric patients. Moreover, the therapist may be the first recipient of clients' erotic fantasies. Sexually provocative behavior toward the therapist, she said, may mask feelings of neediness or rage. The therapist can use individual transferences to facilitate the development of a group identity and peer interaction.

Among many cultures, sexual contact is believed to have life-prolonging or invigorating effects.

> Although movement therapy offers no encompassing solutions for solving the sexual frustrations of the infirm aged, it does offer opportunities for structured physical contact, mutual caring, and open discussion. Touching and being touched appear to have a rejuvenating effect of the participants which increases their alertness and responsiveness to others. Movement therapy, by humanizing the environment, provides opportunities for geriatric patients to experience their sexuality more freely.[33]

## Cardiovascular Patients

At the onset of recovery, cardiovascular patients need to learn new coping skills for stress management. They face fears and anxieties provoked by what many experience as a betrayal of their bodies. Dance therapy helps the individual to increase body awareness for self-monitoring, self-pacing, and physiological control. At the same time, cardiac-rehabilitation program goals encompass physical fitness and a reversal of maladaptive habits that contribute to the original problem.

## Institutional Living

Dance therapist L. Schoenfeld leads dance-therapy groups in nursing facilities as a vehicle for patients to escape the limitations of their disabilities, sicknesses, and restrictions. "Although dealing on a primary level with the limitations of the physical self, the space around that self, and the emotions, my patients can escape these limitations through dance . . . . Expression, exercise, catharsis, group recognition, and acceptance are all important goals in the sessions, but I think the rediscovery of the joy of moving in a creative and aesthetic sense has been the greatest reward for their hard efforts,"[34] says Schoenfeld.

She knows she cannot erase the realities of institutional living nor extensively treat individual psychological problems: "What I can do is facilitate a sense of self-worth within each participant despite the necessary compromises in mobility, focus, sightedness, comprehension, and ability to verbalize."

A typical session begins with gentle stretching and deep breathing, usually unaccompanied by music. Participants move their arms upward, downward, out to the sides, forward, back, and in circles. They wiggle their hips, lift their knees, and carefully stretch their legs. Unison clapping, even if only one hand can be used, in differing musical rhythms and moods, and moving in a circle, pairing up, mirroring each other's movements, and creating a conga line to greet those seated and beckon them to join create energy, stimulation, and calming effects.

## Chronic Pain

Clients often benefit from learning through dance therapy to be aware of underlying affective states and how they are manifest in pain. Therapists refocus awareness from painful to pleasurable body functions and provide tension-reduction and relaxation techniques to manage the stressors of ongoing pain.[35] Intense exercise may create an opiate response.

## Adolescents

Teenagers experience profound physiological and psychological changes. They attempt to cope with the stresses of establishing self-identity, parental expectations, peer pressures, value conflicts, confused self-image, low self-esteem, insecure body image, emerging sexuality, poor impulse control, and difficulty in interpersonal relations.[36] Dance therapy provides an outlet for energy and a safe and playful environment in which many areas of conflict can be identified and worked through, and appropriate adult roles and behavior tried out.

## The Visually Impaired

People are often plagued by the stresses of fantasies and fears stemming from their disabilities. Role-playing and acting out dreams through movement may be a coping mechanism for many such fears. Jo Weisbrod, a licensed professional counselor, describes several of her cases.[37] An eleven year old, concerned that his poor vision would prevent him from having friends and being invited to parties, created several imaginary friends to the detriment of his real friendships. Everyone liked him in his make-believe world. In a movement session, he acted out going to a party. There he danced and talked with friends but was also rejected by a girl he liked and became sad. Following this event he began an entire series of "sad" dances and had begun to face his fear and to deal with his sadness.

In another case, a ten-year-old blind girl who was quite outgoing tried to join many of the games and activities of girls on her block. Despite increasing effort, she met with frustration: Her breath became tighter and shallower. She was especially upset that she kept losing the ball or line marker in the games and worried incessantly that if she could lose an object so easily, maybe she would get lost and never be found.

> During this time we had been doing a lot of deep breathing. One day she sat very still and did not speak. I asked her what was going on; she shook her head. I left her alone and after a while she began exaggerated groping motions. She called her mother for help. Her breath quickened. I did not answer because I felt she had to work this one out on her own. I trusted what was a kind of basic strength within her. She started crying and crawling across the floor. Finally she started a deep breathing sequence I had taught her and said, "I am really all by myself. I can find my way on my knees. I am not lost."

A teenage boy had lost one eye as a child and later the sight of the other eye as a result of abuse by violent and angry parents. He feared that someone would approach him and beat him up. The combined efforts of an understanding teacher, a blind volunteer worker, and the therapist in movement sessions helped him develop extremely acute hearing so he could hear someone coming and defend himself. The DMT sessions focused on moving aggressively so that he developed his physical and psychic strengths until he could protect himself.

A girl who had lost the sight of one eye and had poor vision in the other feared that birds would come and pluck out her one useful eye. Through playing the role of the birds, then of her good eye, and finally of herself, she learned self-protection by shouting and striking out with her arms at the birds.

A forty-year-old totally blind woman institutionalized for additional emotional problems was unable to initiate movement and tended to stand still and to be overcooperative. Dance therapy helped the woman to get "in touch with her own movement so that she could spontaneously reach out and use space around her in a larger, freer way."[38]

## Allied to DMT

### Community-Building with Refugee Children

Allison Jane Singer describes how psychologists and teachers in a nongovernmental organization (NGO) offered multimedia community-building workshops for Serbian refugees and internally displaced children who arrived at a refugee site from different parts of former Yugoslavia during the war between 1991 and 2001.[39] The children faced stresses such as having witnessed violence; migration; resettlement; gaining access to food, housing, education, transport, sanitation, and medical facilities; and feeling disempowerment and dependency. The NGO believes refugee children and families have resources within themselves and within their communities, "hidden voices and treasures," that can be "activated." A way to draw out these resources was through workshops and activities that often included movement as well as other arts (drawing, painting, collage, story making, song) and games. Sometimes attended by up to four hundred people, the workshops were held at the NGO offices, local cultural centers, galleries, museums, parks, and at temporary housing. The NGO asserted that the workshops were *not* therapy targeting specific emotional or psychological problems, but a way to promote social interaction and a new life. Singer observed DM was intrinsic to play and story development as a medium of communication and expression that embodied images, ideas, memories, and emotions. Psychologists did work with individuals on problems that came to the fore in the workshop.

### Support Groups

Related to DMT approaches are types of dance that may provide a supportive group within which to explore negative emotions, to tap unsuspected resources to cope, to express both aloneness and connection, and to remain an individual and yet identify with a group. Some amateur and small professional dance groups, dance-education programs, and DM therapists provide a supportive network. Liz Lerman and her Dance Exchange company of professionals and amateurs helped to pioneer the community residency and community-based art activity to deal with current topics on people's minds. Within the wellness model, contact improvisation (discussed in chapter 9) has a social component of developing trust in another person through a mutual taking and giving of weight, falling, and rolling. The pleasant stimulus of touch in social interaction triggers the release of the powerful peptide hormone oxytocin, which originates in the hypothalamus deep within the brain. Oxytocin does more than create a psychological bond that appears to ward off some of the physical as well as psychological ill effects of stress. It also lowers blood pressure, heart rate, and cortisol levels for up to several weeks, exerting a calming influence.

A culturally based dance-education program for a group of Siouan American Indian female students appeared to be an effective mode of stress reduction for environmental, intrapsychic, and interpersonal stressors. Environmental factors were insecurities about future career plans, financial status, difficulty with academic work, and problems related to living on and/or off the reservations. Intrapsychic issues were health problems such as weight, smoking excessively, alcohol abuse, lack of exercise, as well as feelings about the self and college life. Interpersonal factors were marital status, parenting, family difficulties, being a single parent, meeting their own as well as others' expectations for their role in family and society, and lack of a support system at school.[40]

Former ballroom-dancing champion Taliat Tarsinov says, "When I teach a couple ballroom dancing, I tell them it will be a reflection of life. I will teach you how to lead and follow, how to give each other space so everybody will feel comfortable, how to be next to each other but not in the way of each other."[41]

Some medical doctors teach Middle Eastern dance (belly dance) to women who are stressed about being unable to conceive a child. In the camel move, the breasts at the helm move forward as the buttocks thrusts outward, the stomach contracts, and then the step repeats to vivify the internal organs and to ease uterine fibroids. Isolation of muscle groups moves the upper torso in rotation against a still pelvis or vice versa. Legs rapidly flex and extend to vibrate the hips, and shoulders shimmy. Besides relieving stress, these movements also build physical fitness.

In the late 1980s, circuit parties emerged as a response to the devastation of AIDS. The parties were intended to be an escape through dancing and socializing. Annually, more than fifty events, sometimes lasting day and night over several days, drew an estimated 100,000 gay men during the 1990s.[42] In 1988, Anna Halprin, renowned dancer and choreographer, opened STEPS Theater Company in San Francisco's Firehouse Theater. She gave a weekly four-hour movement workshop for eighteen people who had tested positive for HIV. Participants drew visualizations of their feelings and then embodied them. Halprin's philosophy is that "AIDS is a crisis of the body and it's vital that the body speak its own language, the language of movement, in confronting it."[43] She believes that acting out and physically exploring their illnesses allows participants to bolster their immunological defenses. One workshop, "Circle the Earth: Dancing with Life on the Line," engaged individuals confronting AIDS, their caregivers, and supporters. Over a hundred participants, few of whom had any dance training, explored through movement personal and collective myths about life and death. Halprin and fifteen to twenty HIV-infected participants then created an ongoing performance-oriented group for the men to try to confront their sense of helplessness and fear of the biological and social disease for themselves, those they love, and those they have lost or are about to lose. The video called *Positive Motion*[44] records the first public dance performance, *Carry Me Home*. It shows the ambiguity of defeat and dependence versus triumph and camaraderie. The individuals rediscover their body, alienated from themselves by a virus and politics alike, and experience community as healing.

### Somatic Practices

Somatic practices, also called somatic work, body work, hands-on work, and body-mind disciplines, influenced by Eastern philosophy emerged in the 1970s. These practices help people focus on subtle movement shifts that allow them to correct their choices about how to move in more efficient and integrated ways. The focus is on exploring your anatomy and physiology through the experience of perception and moving. Individuals with health-rehabilitation needs are assisted. Dancers learn to pay attention to their internal mind/body processes while facing the demands of an externally prescribed dance form. Karen Bowes-Sewell, a former ballet dancer who is now a ballet teacher and Feldenkrais practitioner, summarizes some popular body therapies: "The Alexander Technique focuses on the crucial relationship of the head and spine; Ideokinesis harnesses the power of mental imagery to improve movement; Bartenieff Fundamentals™ focuses on integrating efficient movement supported by human developmental patterns; Rolfing works with soft tissue manipulation and movement education to organize the whole body in gravity; Body Mind Centering™ develops a sensory awareness of body tissues and their relationship to expression through movement; and the Feldenkrais Method uses movement and attention as the means for improving our natural abilities to learn, to change and to grow."[45]

A physicist, mechanical engineer, and judo master, Moshe Feldenkrais (1904–1984) developed his somatic approach in response to a debilitating knee injury. He sought to improve the building blocks of human movement found in early childhood development. Bowes-Sewell says, "Feldenkrais work

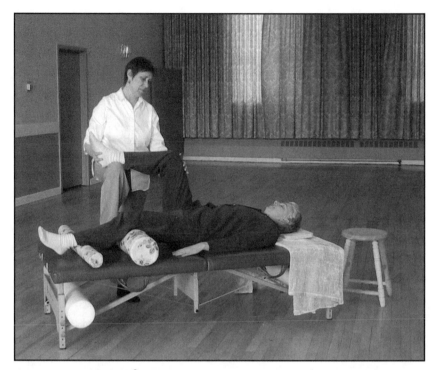

**Figure 11.5.    Feldenkrais® Practitioner Karen Bowes-Sewell with Client (Photo by Karen Bowes-Swell)**

can help to balance the artist's experience by clarifying the sense of self through focused awareness, personal exploration and discovery in a non-competitive situation. I see this as a way to improve the dancer's resilience and ability to thrive in the demanding environment of dance training and performance. With access to more resources within the dancer, I find that the dancer can support the creative process more fully."

## Afterword

DMT bears resemblances to the therapeutic stress-management dance practices found throughout history and non-Western cultures, past and present. Therapists are akin to shamans and other healers. The DMT group-support approach is common, for humans tend to address problems communally. Like DMT, many cultures provide adolescents with dance outlets for various stresses. While DMT appears to have derived from early ritual practices, the various DMT theories may, in fact, illuminate practices of other cultures.

There are a multiplicity of theories, techniques, and clients involved in Western dance therapy. The field is relatively new, but it seems to be increasingly accepted in a host of settings worldwide by health practitioners[46] and the general public. This development coincides with the 1960s awareness of the body and research literature on nonverbal communication that has developed primarily by psychologists since World War II.

In professional dance and, to a lesser extent, amateur dance, the choreographer/dancer chooses to communicate with an audience, be it paying spectators in a theater, a potential sexual partner in a club, or a teacher in a studio. By contrast, for the client in DMT who gives expression to subjective emotion, the therapist or other patients may or may not be relevant receivers of danced messages. The symbolism in any kind of dance, however, allows for recall, reenactment, and reexperience of events for purposes of resisting, reducing, transforming, and escaping stress.

~

# Dance and Stress Resistance, Reduction, and Euphoria

To dance is human. The configuration of human behavior that is called dance has its roots in phylogeny (development of the living species) and ontogeny (development of the individual). Humans have predispositions to dance that are shaped by cultural values and social experience. The physical, affective, and cognitive properties of dance described in the introduction suggest its potential in promoting health and healing. Although there are few statistically based and analyzed control studies that demonstrate specific relationships between dance and stress, compelling theory, supportive case material, and some stand-alone studies exist. However, it is the persistence of dance in helping people to resist, reduce, and escape stress since early humanity that attests to its efficacy.

## Why Dance?

There is no question that there are many ways of dealing with stress. Some are passive activities, such as meditation, yoga, repetitive prayer, biofeedback, or progressive muscle relaxation, that break the train of everyday thought and decrease the activity of the sympathetic nervous system. Other ways of managing stress are active. Exercise has been shown to have long-term effects in developing physical fitness, providing outlets for pent-up tension, reducing anxiety, and developing higher tolerance levels for stress. Exercise utilizes the potentially harmful biochemical elements of energy that are released into the body when it mobilizes against stress in the fight-or-flight response and the individual is in a situation where this energy must be contained. Physical

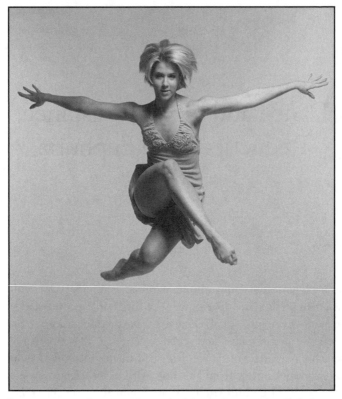

**Figure F.1.   Joy of Dance (Photo of Adrienne Canterna by Chris Dame)**

fitness abets a positive state of mental health that helps you to resist disease. As with many health problems, it is less costly in time, money, and effort to prevent the disabling effects of stress than to arrest or cure them.

If you select an active mode as part of your repertoire of stress-management techniques, why choose dance over other forms of physical exercise? Activities that maintain cardiovascular fitness mainly contract muscles. However, selected forms of dancing provide muscle contraction and stretching as well. Yet dance is more than physical exercise for fitness and movement satisfaction. Dance also permits emotional, intellectual, and aesthetic exploration. Imagination takes reign. A kinetic discourse directed by similar cognitive processes that operate in verbal language, dance is commonly a means of communication, symbolic visualizations embodied in a dancer engaged in self-mastery. Dance often expresses awareness that lacks words. A vehicle that incorporates inchoate ideas in visible human form, dance can modify inner experience and social action. Sometimes dance also allows mastery over others, holding the self and/or the world up to critical scrutiny and shaping one or the other in a desired manner. Dancers' kinetic narratives and poems may confront and work through stressful situations for themselves and empathetically for viewers. Dance releases energy mobilized by the fight-or-flight stress response that was otherwise restrained. Performers' moving images often pay tribute to human fortitude in expressing the sense of doing something and being in control, whether or not a situation can be changed. The discourse of dance can portray human failings and frailties and recount history, make it less traumatic or give it a different outcome. Of course, dance is entertainment that permits diversion and escape from stressors.

A medium for the secular mediation of stress, dance is also a mode of spirituality (personal experience toward connection with the numinous) or religiosity (experience of organized religion) that helps order one's life. Moreover, we know that health care and curing are inseparable from the total history of communal organization and of economy. Stress-related disease may not be only an individual affliction but also a malady that emerges from unfavorable social conditions. The dance may be a vehicle for manifesting divinity and a bringing together of family and community, in reality or fantasy. Additionally, dance is usually accompanied by music, which offers people gratification and functions in ways similar to dance.

Dance is not a single entity or universal medium of communication, but a variety of languages and dialects that work in manifold ways for different kinds of participants. You can be an amateur, a professional dancer, or a client in a dance-therapy situation. Furthermore, a cross-cultural perspective reveals an infinite variety of corporeal techniques. Sometimes dance triggers stress that enables you to deal with greater stressors; at other times, dance is calming. Some people enter trance while dancing; others dance to extricate themselves from trance when a deity incarnates itself within their bodies as vessels. No single explanation fits all dance-stress connections.

In spite of its benefits, dance may not be appropriate for everyone. Some individuals have strong negative attitudes toward dance because of religious training or social upbringing, traumatic experience in dance, or association of dance with specific gender roles or orientation. Physical limitations may also counterindicate dancing. Using dance to discharge tension or escape stress through altered states of consciousness could preclude or retard the resolution of a problem.

For success in avoiding or reducing stress by dancing, you must decide that dance is important. Hopefully this book has convinced you. Which kind of dance provides the greatest benefit is unclear. Much depends upon you and your own mind, body, daily activity, dance instruction, society, and culture. For example, to avoid or reduce stress, professional dancers do supplementary dance exercise outside the studio and theater to enhance their fitness and endurance, which ameliorate the fatigue experienced after several hours of dance-technique classes followed by rehearsal and performance and make dancers less vulnerable to injuries.

## Physical Guideposts

Much of what doctors prescribe for exercise in health and disease generally applies to dance. Paradoxically, the pursuit of good health through exercise may result in injury and impaired health. However, research directs us to ways to make dancing less risky and influence the success of dance in a stress-management program.[1]

Your physical fitness and age are certainly important in selecting the appropriate level for a dance program and the rate of progression. It is critical to take into account your medical history and risk for coronary artery disease. It is useful for a sedentary person to have a medical examination with stress tests (e.g., treadmill, bicycle, and step) before embarking upon a dance program. Dancing for older adults requires special care because of the dire medical consequences of physical stress.[2] Heart patients need to be aware that beta endorphins, the opiumlike pain-killing brain chemicals associated with exhilaration and the runner's high, could hide symptoms of dangerous heart damage. It is preferable that heart patients feel the stress on their hearts so that they can reduce their activity if necessary.

For the nonprofessional, beginning a dance program gradually and using moderation are keys to preventing physical harm. Aerobic exercise from three to five days per week with conditioning every other day is recommended for fitness. A regimen of dance coupled with rest time between workouts for the musculoskeletal system to adapt is most likely to build endurance and prevent injury. This pattern provides immediate physical reinforcement as well as long-term benefit.

The climatic environment in which professionals or amateurs dance influences their ability to perform successfully. High temperature, humidity, and radiation from the sun combined with low air movement and lack of dancer acclimatization put stress on the dancer if the movement is intense and of long duration. If a person does not drink water or a diluted electrolyte solution for quick rehydration, dehydration—body-water loss from exercising in the heat—can result in heat exhaustion or stroke. Since dancing itself creates considerable body heat on top of that provided by the dancer's clothing, moving in cooler settings allows you to avoid these problems. The body does take a longer time to warm up in cooler settings, however. In certain areas of the United States, air pollution, especially high concentrations of carbon monoxide and ozone, can have a negative effect on any exercise. When pollution reaches the "air alert" stage, no exercise is recommended. People unaccustomed to high altitudes find their bodies have difficulty delivering oxygen to working muscles, and thus movement capacity diminishes. Floor surfaces should have resilience (wood or special composition) for dancing in order to prevent leg and back injuries.

Clothing and shoes make a difference. Over- or underdressing, or wearing the wrong size or type of shoe, can cause climatic stress, disability, or injury. Doctors say that under no circumstances should you exercise while wearing rubberized or plastic clothing, because it does not allow body sweat to evaporate. Through sweating the body regulates its temperature during exercise, and reduced evaporation of sweat can dramatically increase body temperature, dehydration, and salt loss.[3]

Some dance, such as modern and Afro-Caribbean, calls for bare feet. Until the bottoms of their feet toughen and develop protective calluses, beginners may develop blisters. A toe box in any shoe with insufficient clearance between the toes and the underside of the toe box may cause black toenails as a result of the formation of blood blisters under the toenail. Tap, jazz, ballet, and toe shoes require proper fitting, which can usually be obtained in specialized dance-supply stores. For example, leather jazz shoes are at first supposed to feel very tight since the soft leather stretches as you dance. For aerobics dancing, a shoe with good shock-absorbing qualities and lateral support is desirable.

Blisters resulting from dancing with tender feet or new shoes should be punctured at the edge with a sterile needle to drain the fluid and then covered with a topical antiseptic and bandage. Muscle cramps, involuntary muscle contractions that are possibly the result of a salt and potassium imbalance in the muscle, can be relieved with stretching and massage. For bone bruises on the bottoms of the feet caused by jumping or leaping, ice and padding on the area provide some relief. Knee pain and shin splits (a sharp pain on the front of the tibia, probably due to factors such as a lowered arch, hairline or stress fracture of the bone, or tearing of the muscle where it attaches to bone) usually respond to rest. Immediately icing an injury and taking an anti-inflammatory drug tend to prevent major swelling.

A dance session, class, or activity should begin with a warm-up, preferably until the body begins to perspire. Sudden vigorous exercise places a potentially lethal strain on the heart. Stretching exercises after the body is warm help to develop and maintain flexibility in addition to preparing the muscles, joints, and ligaments for dancing. And after dancing, a cool-down helps to prevent bodily injury such as muscle pulls, strains, sprains, and lower-back discomfort, as well as reducing the extent of muscle soreness. Walking or similar locomotion in an upright position can prevent blood from pooling in the lower half of the body and allow the leg muscles to assist the return of any pooled blood to the heart, which, in turn, provides an adequate blood flow to the brain. Abrupt stopping of vigorous dancing and inadequate blood flow to the brain could cause you to become dizzy and even pass out. Following a dance workout, a warm, rather than a hot, shower is recommended. The latter can create the cardiovascular complications of peripheral dilation and blood pooling.

Dancers need to be aware of signals from their bodies in order to avoid physical stress, injury, and even death. They should have realistic expectations about what they can do within a given period of time, the constraints of body build, such as a pelvic structure that precludes a 180 degree turn out at the hip joint, or an inefficient cardiovascular system, and prior experience. Suffering previous injuries alerts one to potential weaknesses and recurrence. Alas, living past the age of thirty-five means that there is a chance of bodily wear and tear in parts of the body predisposing them to a breakdown with overexertion. If you have a vulnerable area, massage or warm water will loosen the muscles and increase the blood supply.

Warning signs and discomfort may occur either during, immediately after exercise, or up to forty-eight hours later; as is the case for jogging.[4] Abnormal heart activity (irregular pulse, either a sudden burst of rapid heartbeats or a slow pulse falling rapidly); pain or pressure in the chest, arm, or throat; sudden lack of coordination, confusion; cold sweating; pallor; a purplish discoloration of the skin due to deficient oxygenation of the blood; and fainting indicate you should stop dancing and see a physician before resuming exercise. Dancing should be avoided when fever is present, since viral infections can possibly infect the heart muscle.

Some symptoms call for corrective measures to prevent injury. If such problems do not disappear with remedial action, then a physician consultation is appropriate. For a rapid pulse rate that persists for five to ten minutes of recovery or longer, you should reduce the intensity of dancing and progress to higher levels of dance activity at a slower rate. Nausea or vomiting after dancing may require a reduced intensity and a prolonged cool-down period as well as avoidance of eating for at least two hours prior to dancing. Extreme breathlessness lasting more than ten minutes after you stop dancing and prolonged fatigue up to twenty-four hours after exercise may respond to a reduction in the intensity of dancing.

Some individuals are strongly habituated to dancing that brings about a good feeling, energy, and productivity. This dance program works for them most of the time. However, when an accident occurs that prevents the customary dancing, the individual (as I experienced after an accident that kept me immobile for a time) may experience more stress than otherwise.

In selecting a dance-therapy program, it is important to have a trained instructor/therapist who understands kinesiology and is sensitive to your needs. Sometimes teachers teach what they were taught or what works for their own bodies even though it contradicts contemporary knowledge about healthy practice.

Dancers need to be aware of the danger of excessive thinness and vigorous exercise. As noted earlier, this combination disrupts the menstrual cycle, lowers estrogen levels, endangers fertility, decreases the body's ability to utilize calcium, interferes with bone-mineral content, and increases the risk of bone injury.

## Cognitive Counsel

The level of dance activity you undertake has implications for stress. Selection of dance activities that are too simple may lead to boredom. Activities that are demanding tend to be regarded as stimulating and energizing. However, if they are too demanding they may tax your coping ability and elicit high levels of anxiety and reduced effort, fatigue, exhaustion, and burnout. If you do not like one class or teacher (personality, selection of music, or style of instruction), try another. Experiment with different forms of dance and varying levels of difficulty.

Dancers can draw upon a variety of techniques to cope with performance anxiety and fear and to improve performance, which, in turn, often decreases stage fright. Biofeedback helps you assess your own internal stress responses through, for example, muscle tension, skin temperature, sweat activity, elevated heart rate, and dry mouth. Meditation techniques such as transcendental meditation (TM), yoga, and Zen tend to induce relaxation before a performance and to promote improved concentration for body control. Positive thinking and autogenics involve verbalizing and visualizing a desired outcome so that performance anxiety is allayed.

Imagery (formerly known as mental practice) refers to visualizing oneself performing a skill or entire choreography and rehearsing it in one's mind prior to its actual execution. There is either a mental image in our brain, or the graphic and detailed nature of language makes it seem so. Imaging a dance action initiates electrical impulses along certain neurological pathways to the musculature involved in the movement, thus activating it and inhibiting impulses to other muscles. There are two kinds of imagery. Internal imagery is your imagination of the kinesthetic experience of the correct performance of a movement. External imagery is the visualization of yourself performing the movement.

Visual-motor behavior rehearsal (VMBR) combines relaxation and imagery. Going through stressful experiences mentally should make it easier to deal with the stress of actual performance. Body therapies, in which you draw upon the visualization of accurate images of intended movements, are a way to augment injury-prevention activities as well as rehabilitation between the end of medical treatment and the return to skilled performance.[5] The Alexander technique, Ashton patterning, bioenergetics, Bonnie Cohen's Mind/Body Centering, Feldenkrais awareness through movement, Jacobson's progressive relaxation, Laban/Bartenieff movement analysis, Rolfing integration of human structure, Silver's sensory awareness, Todd/Sweigard ideokinetic facilitation, and Trager psychophysical integration are some of the therapy principles and interventions available to dancers. They attempt to draw awareness to maladaptive automatic-motor habits in order to discover new and more-effective patterns of, for example, body alignment, breathing patterns, and mechanical balance.

## Finding Meaning in Movement

Meaning in dance depends on who does what, when, where, why, how, and with and to whom. Such variables can convey gender roles, social-class status hierarchies, race, and other group identities. A semantic grid is a useful tool for understanding meaning in movement for dance therapy (in diagnosing problems, measuring change, and interpreting client insights mediated through dance) and for observers of dance in exotic societies or their own theaters. I developed this tool in trying to discover meaning in Nigeria's Ubakala Igbo dance and analyze it in cross-cultural perspective. Subsequently, I have used it in my other dance studies. Although there are several notation systems that describe movements as motion, none refers to what the movements signify or offers direction in identifying such meaning. Meaning is communication in contexts with shared understanding among dancers and observers. You may find meaning in dance irrespective of what the dancer intends to communicate. Meaning may lie in the rules dictating how signs may be combined, that is, the grammar; a different way of saying something (how) may be saying a different thing (what).

To probe for meaning, the grid can be imposed on the whole dance and used to zoom in on smaller units as you would turn a telescope lens in order to bring images into focus. Placing each unit of dance within each cell of the grid matrix permits considering the possibility (existence or nonexistence) of forms of encoding meaning and the transformation of these over time.

Let us turn to the grid (which should be read vertically). Six devices that have been found in a global survey of dance are presented for conveying meaning. Each device may be conventional (customary shared legacy) or autographic (idiosyncratic or creative expression of a thing, event, or condition). (1) A *concretization* produces the outward aspect of a thing, event, or condition, for example, mimetically portraying a battle. It is an imitation. (2) An *icon* represents most properties of a thing, event, or condition and is responded to as if it were what it represents. An example is dancing the role of a deity who is revered or otherwise treated as the deity. The Haitians believe Ghede appears when a dancer is possessed by him, and they treat the dancer in this state with genuine awe. (3) A *stylization* encompasses somewhat arbitrary gestures or movements that are the result of convention. In ballet, pointing to the heart is a sign of love. (4) A *metonym is* a motional conceptualization of one thing for that of another of which it is an attribute or extension. A war dance as part of a battle is a case in point. (5) A *metaphor* expresses one thought, experience, or phenomenon in place of another that resembles the former to suggest an analogy between the two. Dancing the role of a leopard to denote the power of death is an example. (6) An *actualization* is an individual dancing one or several of his usual statuses and roles, such as Louis XIV dancing the role of king and being treated as such.

Meaning usually depends on context. The devices for encapsulating meaning seem to operate within one or more of eight spheres: (1) the event and/or situation, (2) the total human body in action, (3) the whole pattern of the performance, (4) the discursive aspect of the performance (the sequence of unfolding movement configurations), (5) specific movement, (6) the intermeshing of movement with other communication media (for example, dance meaning being inseparable from song, music, costume, accoutrement, and/or speech), (7) dance movement as a vehicle for another medium (for example, dance providing background for a performer's poetry recitation), and (8) presence (the emotional turn-on through projected sensuality or charisma).

Singly or in combination, these devices and spheres allow you to probe for messages. The devices are signs that may function as signals when they are directly related to the action they signify, such as a war dance to herald a battle. Other relevant considerations are how movers use movement and relate to each other in the process, what the movers and observers say about

| Devices | Spheres | | | | | | | |
|---|---|---|---|---|---|---|---|---|
| | Event | Body in Action | Whole Performance | Discursive Performance | Specific Movement | Intermesh with other Media | Vehicle for other Medium | Presence |
| Concretization | | | | | | | | |
| Icon | | | | | | | | |
| Stylization | | | | | | | | |
| Metonym | | | | | | | | |
| Metaphor | | | | | | | | |
| Actualization | | | | | | | | |

Figure F.2. Dimensions of Meaning in Dance

the movement, and how movement symbols relate to other symbols used by the individual and by her or his society. It is important to consider the tacit knowledge, hierarchical levels of meaning, use of opposites and inversions, ambiguity, synonyms, changing meaning of a device at different phases in performance, and operation of metaphoric equations in two directions at once. Illustratively, if one is dancing Dylan Thomas's "Our Eunuch Dreams," one needs to know not only that a eunuch is a man who has been castrated but also that castration destroys sexual potency, and that sexual potency is to be taken as a symbol of efficacy in general. Saying the lion is king of the beasts says something about lions and also something about kings.

## Afterword

I have explored patterns of dance and stress, how dance may be a means through which people resist, reduce, induce, and escape stress as well as become euphoric. The journey has encompassed a broad view of past and present and near and far cultures to reveal a kaleidoscopic variety and complexity in the human dance repertoire. Through dance, people meet demons, ward off death, shake off sin and evil, come to terms with life crises, mediate paradoxes, resolve conflict, revitalize the past to re-create the present, enhance their self-concept and body image, attract attention, assert themselves, confront the strong, and persuade others to change their ways. Every society attempts to define stress and to explain its causes and proper responses. When social conflict causes stress, effective dance therapy tends to be group-related with an interpersonal script. Danced healing rituals (in African village compounds, temple courtyards, dance-therapy studios, public theaters, and other social settings) reinvoke old traumas for exorcism and the transformation of fear, convince people that evil is gone or possible to dissipate, and reaffirm communal solidarity and a sense of well-being. Disclosure of problems through personal introspection, masked demon dancing or other supernatural revelation is to expose problems to therapeutic action. Dance is frequently part of a group's roots, something that belongs to them. Whether manifest in Zulu mobilization for war or American marathon defense against the Depression, dance often has an affective contagion.

In the interweave of mind and body, dance is a mode that allows people to work through difficulties, anticipate the future, recollect the past, and confront the present. Participants in dance, both dancers and viewers, may experience catharsis and develop a sense of mastery or self-discovery. Moreover, movers may achieve physical fitness, which ameliorates fatigue, aging, premenstrual discomfort, and disease. Be it tarantism or contemporary amateur or professional theater art, the dance medium gives scope for self-expression and opportunity for approbation.

In sum, dance may be pleasurable in and of itself; however, dance also moves individuals to personal and social action beyond the dance setting. Prophylactic against the negative affects of stress and remediative in transforming distress, dance has unique potential. It is my hope that this book will stimulate further exploration in connections between dance and stress in order to generate knowledge that will help people better cope with stress in modern society and attain an exquisite balance of being. In the United States and other countries, there has been a decline in public and private support of the arts, including dance. Awareness that dance is not just entertainment but also a form of education and healing may reverse the trend.

~

# Notes

## Prelude

1. Samuels 2001; McNally 2003; Myers 2003.
2. Carlson 2004, 16.
3. Nichter and Lock 2002.
4. See Hanna 1970, 1978, 1983, 1987b, 1988c, 1990, 1995, 1999. I have served on the editorial board of the *American Journal of Dance Therapy* since 1988.
5. Hoge et al. 2004.
6. Cohen-Sandler 2005.
7. Christakis and Allison 2006.
8. Marmot 2004; Schwartz 2004.
9. Laufer 2003.
10. Schwartz 2004.
11. McDonald 1998.
12. Vogel 1986.
13. Reid 2003.
14. Baker 2004.
15. Wampold 2001.
16. Fox 1999; Jackson et al. 2004.
17. Nieman 1998, 253.
18. Squires 2001; see Dunn et al. 2005; Stein 2005; and Moffet et al. 2002.
19. McDonald 1998.
20. Yamaguchi 2000.
21. Hanna 1982, 1986b, 1988b.
22. Hanna 1983.

## Chapter 1

1. Selye 1974, 1976.
2. McEwen 2002. See also Toates 1995; Turner, Wheaton, and Lloyd 1995; Sapolsky 2004.
3. Morley and Morimoto 2004.
4. See Sapolsky 1992, 2004; Avison 1994.
5. Damasio 2003.
6. McEwen 2002, 9.
7. McElroy and Townsend 1979.
8. Friedman 2003.
9. See Lovallo 1997; Lazarus 1999; Payne and Cooper 2001.
10. Cole 2003.

11. Wilson et al. 2003.
12. Cannon 1929, 1932.
13. Quoted in Zimmerman 2003.
14. Selye 1976.
15. See Mackinnon 1992; Wittstein et al. 2005; and Yusuf et al. 2004 on the relationship between anger and angina problems.
16. McEven 2002, 36–37.
17. Brewin 2003.
18. Brewin 2003, 193.
19. Brewin 2003, 203.
20. Duke 2004.
21. See McEwen 2002 and Sapolsky 2004 for copious references.
22. Rosenkranz et al. 2005.
23. Wang et al. 2004.
24. Epel et al. 2004.
25. See Hanna references.
26. Cooper 1970.
27. See Tipton 2003.
28. Raglin 1997; Martinsen et al. 1997.
29. Csikszentmihalyi 1975.
30. Quoted in Gruen 1986, 33.
31. Insel, Gingrich, and Young 2001.
32. Heinrichs 2003.
33. McEwen 2002, 173.
34. Insel, Gingrich, and Young 2001.
35. Graham 1985.
36. Hackney 2000.
37. Douglas 1970, 1973.
38. Gardner 1983.

## Chapter 2

1. Lawler 1964.
2. Roth 1998.
3. Paffenbarger Jr. 1986.
4. Verghese 2003; Coyle 2003.
5. Smith and Serfass 1981, 179; Montoye 1984.
6. Wilson et al. 2003.
7. Verghese et al. 2003.
8. Scheff 1977.
9. Serlin 1985.
10. Frank 1973, 318. Mental illness is conceptualized as the breakdown in an individual's adaptation to the environment that creates subjective distress and objective disability, disharmony within persons and between them and their societies, and the expression of disorders of communication based on past experience.
11. Lambo 1965.
12. Snyder 2001.
13. Catlin 2004.
14. Catlin, personal communication; see Barnes 1992.
15. Munroe 1955, 630.
16. Berger 1984, 139.
17. Griaule 1965, 188.
18. Safier 1953, 242; Morgan 1984, 142.
19. Lamb 1978, 283.
20. Morgan 1985, 96.
21. Sachs and Buffone 1984.
22. Hanna 1983.
23. K. White 2006.
24. Gottschild 2003.
25. See O'Connor and Shimizu 2002 for a comparison of British and Japanese cultural value systems.
26. Ho 2005.
27. Farrer 1976.
28. Madsen 1973, 1989–1996.
29. Fergusson 1931, xxi.
30. Hanna 1987a; 1987b, chap. 5; 1988c.
31. Hoerburger 1965.
32. Kealiinohomoku 1969–1970.
33. Rovner 1986.

## Chapter 3

1. Horton 1960.
2. Ten Raa 1969.
3. Drewal 1992.
4. Rigby 1966.
5. Akstein 1973.
6. Sangree 1969, 1,055.
7. Kendall 1985.
8. Crapanzano 1973, 195–210, 231–34.
9. McElroy and Townsend 1979, 295.
10. Laderman 1996.
11. Laderman 1996, 137.
12. Roseman 1991, 2002.
13. Marshall 1969, 12; Lee 1967.
14. McElroy and Townsend 1979, 277.
15. Guenther 1975, 162.
16. Guenther 1975.
17. Williams 1974.
18. Tamuno 1966.
19. Chilivumbo 1969.
20. Williams 1968.
21. Kapferer 1983.
22. Kapferer 1983, 108.
23. Kapferer 1983, 106.
24. Kapferer 1983, 151.
25. Kapferer 1983, 183.
26. Kapferer 1983, 50.
27. Kapferer 1983, 62.
28. Kapferer 1983, 71.
29. Kapferer 1983, 177.
30. Kapferer 1983, 192.
31. Kapferer 1983, 229.

## Chapter 4

1. Russell 1979.
2. Hecker 1885, 73.
3. Rouget 1985.
4. Quoted in De Martino 1966, 385.
5. De Martino 1966, 68–73.
6. De Martino 1966, 160.
7. De Martino 1966, 214–15.
8. Rouget 1986, 159.
9. Schneider 1948.
10. Rouget 1985, 159.
11. De Martino 1966, 304.
12. De Martino 1966, 240.
13. Rouget 1986, 164–65.
14. Benedictow 2004, 393.
15. Hecker 1885; Benedictow 2004.
16. Kelly 2005.
17. Backman 1952.
18. McKean 1979.
19. Kern 1981.
20. See Shorter 1982.
21. Kern 1987, 74.
22. Kern 1981, 100; Andrews 1940, 144–45.

## Chapter 5

1. Hanna 1986b.
2. Hanna 1989.
3. Hanna and Hanna 1968.
4. Wolpe 1958.
5. Freud 1955, 14–17.
6. Bychowski 1951, 393.
7. Okonkwo 1971, 149.
8. Cf. Keleman 1975.
9. See Uchendu 1965, 12.
10. Umunna 1968, 28.
11. Ottenberg and Ottenberg 1964, 31.
12. Ottenberg and Ottenberg 1964, 31.
13. Ilogu 1965, 338.
14. Safier 1953, 242.

15. Nwoga 1971, 34.
16. Spencer 1985.
17. Spencer 1985, 155.
18. Spencer 1985, 145.
19. Spencer 1985, 147–48.
20. Spencer 1985, 144–45.

21. Spencer 1985, 147.
22. Middleton 1985, 166.
23. Middleton 1985, 167.
24. Wilson 1954.
25. Griaule 1965.

## Chapter 6

1. Schechner 1973, 33.
2. See Frank 1973, 318.
3. Turner 1974.
4. Gailey 1970 provides one of the fullest accounts.
5. Njaka 1974, 22.
6. Van Allen 1972, Dorward 1982.
7. City Ordinance 591/2, quoted in Nwabara 1965, 188–89.
8. Meek 1937, 201.

9. Nwabara 1965, 231.
10. Perham 1937, 208.
11. See Nigerian Government 1930a and 1930b; Perham 1937, 206–20; Onwuteaka 1965.
12. Cf. Hanna 1988a.
13. Hanna 1982, 1986a, 1988b.
14. Hansen 1967; Levine 1977.
15. Jones and Hawes 1972, 124.
16. Jones and Hawes 1972, 67–68.

## Chapter 7

1. Fernandez 1982.
2. Fernandez 1982, 571.
3. Fernandez 1982, 4.
4. Fernandez 1982, 562.
5. Fernandez 1982, 566.
6. Fernandez 1982, 305.
7. Fernandez 1982, 532.
8. Fernandez 1982, 389.
9. Fernandez 1982, 417.
10. Fernandez 1982, 450.
11. Fernandez 1982, 475.
12. Stewart 1980.

13. Thornton 1981.
14. Mooney 1965, 77.
15. Amoss 1978.
16. Amoss 1978, 45.
17. Howard 1976.
18. Quoted in Howard 1976, 247.
19. See Mitchell 1956 on the Kalela dance in Africa for a similar pattern.
20. Moedano 1972.
21. Ranger 1975.
22. Ranger 1975, 6.

## Chapter 8

1. Quoted in DeNatale 2000.
2. DeNatele 2000.
3. Quoted in Samuels 2001.
4. Yatkin, personal commuinication.
5. Siegel 1977, 178–79.

6. Siegel 1977, 213.
7. Kisselgoff 1982.
8. Siegel 1977, 122–23.
9. Dunning 1986.
10. Roberts 2004.

11. Kriegsman 1987, 10.
12. Dunning 2004.
13. Hanna 1988a.
14. Hanna 1998, 2003, 2005a.
15. Bullough 1976.
16. Jackson 1978, 38.

17. Quoted in Parks 1986, 56.
18. Quoted in Wallach 1989.
19. Gere 2004, 35.
20. Raymond 1979, 104.
21. Brierley 1979.

## Chapter 9

1. Bentley 1986.
2. Hager 1978.
3. Quoted in Thompson 2004.
4. See Hamilton 1997, 1998, 1999; Hamilton and Hamilton 1994, 1995.
5. Shell 1986.
6. Kirkland 1986, 26–27.
7. Kirkland 1986, 212.
8. De Mille 1960, 4.
9. Hanna 1990.
10. Hanna 1998, 2003, 2005a.
11. Quoted in Jowitt 1995.
12. Temin 1982.
13. Quoted in Stoop 1984, 62.
14. *Washington Post* 1980.
15. Gold 2001.
16. Halpern 1981.
17. Braiker 1986.
18. Hanna 1997, 2002b, 2005c.
19. Quoted in Deans 2001, 3.
20. Quoted in Deans 2001, 4.
21. Clark et al. 2005.
22. DeFrantz 2004.
23. Quoted in *Sydney Morning Herald* 2003.
24. Reagan 1983.
25. Chryst 1986, 44.
26. Quoted in Weston 1982, 11.
27. Farrell 1990.
28. Farrell 1990, 28–29.
29. Farrell 1990, 109–10.
30. Kirkland 1986, 50.
31. Kirkland 1986, 45.
32. Kirkland 1986, 48.

33. Kirkland 1986, 68.
34. Kirkland 1986, 67.
35. Kirkland 1986, 118.
36. Kirkland 1986, 175.
37. Kirkland 1986, 90.
38. Kirkland 1986, 244.
39. Kirkland 1986, 40.
40. Kirkland 1986, 41.
41. Quoted in Temin 1982[0].
42. Kirkland 1986, 34.
43. Kirkland 1986, 51.
44. Kirkland 1986, 96.
45. Farrell 1990, 279.
46. Novack 1990.
47. Rockwell 1988.
48. Pierpont 1984.
49. Forsyth and Kolenda 1966; Fishman 2004.
50. Rasta Thomas, personal communication.
51. Hanna 1985, 1988a.
52. Dan Thomas, personal communication.
53. Rasta Thomas, personal communication.
54. Quoted in Jacob 1981, 297.
55. Aaron 1986.
56. Rockwell and Nadel 1984.
57. See Helin 1989.
58. Taylor 1999.
59. See psychoanalyst Sanford Weisblatt in Anon. 1986, 13.
60. Kirkland 1986, 37.
61. Bentley 1982, 6–7.

62. Bentley 1982, 8.
63. Bentley 1982, 12.
64. Bentley 1982, 14.
65. Bentley 1982, 96–99.
66. Bentley 1982, 148–49.
67. Quoted in Jacob 1981, 285.
68. Quoted in Robson and Gillies 1987.
69. White 1982.
70. Rasta Thomas, personal communication.
71. Thompson 2004.
72. Smith, Ptacek, and Patterson 2000.
73. Fonseca, personal communication.
74. Anderson 1985.
75. Vincent 1979.
76. Gordon 1983, 173.
77. Kirkland 1986, 56.
78. See Panov 1978 on stresses unique to dancers in the Soviet Union; Hanna 2004a, 2004b on dance in Cuba.
79. *Washington Post* 1983.
80. McCarthy et al. 2001; Hanna 2002a.
81. Smith 2003.
82. McCarthy and Jinnett 2001, xi.
83. Bentley 1982, 18.
84. Kirkland 1986, 185.
85. Bentley 1982, 64–65.
86. Bentley 1982, 89.
87. Yatkin, personal communication.
88. Quoted in McIntyre 1986.
89. Alliance for the Arts 1985.
90. Dunning 1987.
91. Hanna 1985.
92. Sociologist David Earl Sutherland, quoted in Weston 1982, 11.
93. Solway 1986.
94. Quoted in Weston 1982.
95. Quoted in Jacob 1981, 96.
96. Jacob 1981.
97. Quoted in Kelly-Saxenmeyer 2004.
98. Mazo 1974, 105–6.
99. Quoted in Kirkland 1986, 212.

## Chapter 10

1. Hanna 2004c.
2. Personal communication.
3. Hendin and Csikszentmihalyi 1975, 104–5.
4. Silver 1981.
5. Peiss 1986.
6. Peiss 1986, 110.
7. Martin 1986.
8. Calabria 1976, 57.
9. Quoted in Martin 1986, 16.
10. Quoted in Martin 1986, 14.
11. Quoted in Martin 1986, 7.
12. Quoted in Martin 1986, 17.
13. María Luz Guarrochena quoted in Rohter 2003.
14. Blum 1966–1967.
15. Quoted in Blum 1966–1967, 359.
16. Quoted in Blum 1966–1967, 362.
17. Quoted in Blum 1966–1967, 359.
18. Quoted in Blum 1966–1967, 360.
19. Sommer 1983, 29.
20. Sommer 1983, 31.
21. Sommer 1983, 29.
22. Sommer 1983, 29.
23. Thomas 2003.
24. Jackson 2004, 15.
25. Quoted in Jackson 2004, 23.
26. Hanna 2004d.
27. All quoted in McNees 1987.
28. Lopata and Noel 1972.
29. Lopata and Noel 1972.
30. Lopata and Noel 1972, 188–89.
31. Valleroy, personal communication.
32. Forman 1983.

# Chapter 11

1. Dulicai and Berger 2005.
2. Siegel 1984; Payne 1992; Halpirin 2003; Levy 2005.
3. See *American Journal of Dance Therapy;* Mason 1974; Delaney 1982; Bernstein 1979; Levanthal 1983.
4. Robben and Suárez-Orozco 2002.
5. Brewin 2003.
6. See, e.g., Bernstein 1995; Chang and Leventhal 1995; Frank 1997; Gray 2001.
7. Hutchinson 1961; Dell 1970.
8. Bernstein 1979.
9. Schmais 2004.
10. Serlin 1977, 145.
11. Exiner and Kelynack 1994.
12. Schmais 1985.
13. Schmais 1985, 25.
14. Schmais 1985, 27–28.
15. Schmais 1985, 31.
16. Schmais 1985, 31–32.
17. Schmais 1985, 33–34.
18. Akstein 1973.
19. Rockwell 1988.
20. Manning and Fabrega 1973.
21. Dressor 1996.
22. Sandel 1980.
23. Sandel 1980, 21.
24. Sandel 1980, 31.
25. Plevin 2003.
26. Plevin, personal communication.
27. Berstein 1995.
28. Chang and Leventhal 1995.
29. Eley 2004.
30. Anon. 1979.
31. Verghese et al. 2003; Coyle 2003.
32. Lerman 1984.
33. Verghese et al. 2003; Coyle 2003.
34. Schoenfeld 1986.
35. Perlman et al. 1990.
36. Brown and Lawton 1987.
37. Weisbrod 1974.
38. Weisbrod 1974, 51–52.
39. Singer 2005.
40. Skye, Christensen, and England 1989.
41. Berger 2003.
42. Signorile 1997.
43. Quoted in Ross 1989.
44. Wilson 1991.
45. Bowes-Sewell 2004.
46. Goodill 2005.

# Finale

1. See, e.g., Howes and McCormack 2000; Fitt 1996; Berardi 2005; Solomon, Solomon, and Minton 2005.
2. Smith and Serfass 1981.
3. Pollock et al. 1984, 375.
4. Sachs and Buffone 1984.
5. Meyers 1986; Meyers, Pierpont, and Schnitt 1986.

# References

Aaron, S. 1986. *Stage fright: Its role in acting.* Chicago: University of Chicago Press.

Abrams, G. L. 1985–1986. Report on the First international conference on mind, body and the performing arts: Stress processes in the psychology and physiology of music, dance and drama, New York University, July 15–19, 1985. *Dance Research Journal* 17 (2) and 18 (1).

Adams, C. 1986. Collaboration: An artist's view. *Update Dance/USA* 4 (1): 8.

Akstein, D. 1973. Terpsichoreotrancetherapy: A new hypopsychotherapeutic method. *International Journal of Clinical and Experimental Hypnosis* 21 (3): 131–43.

Alliance for the Arts. 1985. *Spaces for the arts: A study of the real estate needs of non-profit arts organizations in New York City.* New York: Alliance for the Arts.

Amoss, P. 1978. *Coast Salish Spirit Dancing: The survival of an ancestral religion.* Seattle: University of Washington Press.

Anderson, D. 1985. Eating disorders. *Update Dance/USA* 3 (7): 9–11.

Anderson, J. 1986. Dance: D. J. McDonald explores growing old. *New York Times,* February 26, C1.

Andrews, E. A. 1940. *The gift to be simple: Songs, dances and rituals of the American Shakers.* New York: Dover.

Anon. 1979. Stressful living country-style. *Behavioral Medicine* 6 (2): 36–39.

Anon. 1986. Coping with stress: Roundtable discussion. *Medical Problems of Performing Artists.* 1 (1): 12–16.

Avison, W. R., and I. H. Gotlieb, eds. 1994. *Stress and mental health: Contemporary issues and prospects for the future.* New York: Plenum Press.

Backman, E. L. 1952. *Religious dances in the Christian church and in popular medicine.* Trans. E. Classen. London: George Allen and Unwin.

Baker, B. 2004. The art of healing: Visual and performing arts take on a bigger role in patient recovery. *Washington Post,* August 17, F1.

Barnes, C. 1992. Comedy in dance. In *The dance has many faces*, ed. W. Sorrell, 87–95. New York: Pennington/A Cappella.

Benedictow, O. J. 2004. *The Black Death 1346–1353: The complete history*. Woodbridge, UK: Boydell Press.

Ben-Ezra, M. 2002. Trauma 4,000 years ago? *American Psychiatric Association*, 159: 1437.

Bentley, T. 1982. *Winter season: A dancer's journal*. New York: Random House.

———. 1986. Reaching for perfection: The life and death of a dancer. *New York Times*, April 17, H1, 25.

Berardi, G. M. 2005. *Finding balance: Fitness, training, and health for a lifetime in dance*. 2nd ed. New York: Routledge.

Berger, B. G. 1984. Running away from anxiety and depression: A female as well as male race. In *Running as therapy: An integrated approach*, ed. M. L. Sachs and G. W. Buffone, 138–71. Lincoln: University of Nebraska Press.

Berger, J. 2003. The Russians are coming, stepping lightly. *New York Times*, June 11.

Bernstein, P. 1979. *Eight theoretical approaches in dance-movement therapy*. Dubuque, IA: Kendall Hunt.

———. 1995. Dancing beyond trauma: Women survivors of sexual abuse. In *Dance and other expressive art therapies: When words are not enough*, ed. F. J. Levy with J. P. Fried and F. Leventhal, 41–58. New York: Routledge.

Blom, L. A. 1986. What makes a dance funny? *American Dance 2*.

Blum, L. H. 1966–1967. The discotheque and the phenomenon of alone-togetherness! *Adolescence* 1 (4): 351–66.

Bowes-Sewell, K. 2004. The Feldenkrais Method: How can it benefit dancers? *Dance Current*, September, 1, 167.

Braiker, H. 1986. *The type E woman: How to overcome the stress of being everything to everybody*. Nashville, TN: Dodd Mead.

Brewin, C. R. 2003. *Post-traumatic stress disorder: Malady or myth?* New Haven, CT: Yale University Press.

Brierly, H. 1979. *Transvestism*. Oxford: Pergamon Press.

Brown, D. E. 1981. General stress in anthropological fieldwork. *American Anthropologist* 83 (1): 74–92.

Brown, G. K., T. Ten Have, G. Henriques, and A. T. Beck. 2005. Cognitive therapy for the prevention of suicide attempts: A randomized controlled trial. *Journal of the American Medical Association* 294 (5):563–70.

Brown, J. D., and M. Lawton. 1987. Stress and well-being in adolescence: The moderating role of physical exercise. *Journal of Human Stress* 12 (3): 125–31.

Buckroyd, J. 2000. *The student dancer: Emotional aspects of the teaching and learning of dance*. London: Dance Books.

Bychowski, G. 1951. From catharsis to work of art: The making of an artist. In *Psychoanalysis and culture: Essays in honor of Geza Roheim*, ed. G. B. Wilbur and W. Muensterberger, 390–409. New York: International Universities Press.

Calabria, F. M. 1976. The dance marathon craze. *Journal of Popular Culture* 10 (1): 54–69.

Cannon, W. B. 1929. *Bodily changes in pain, hunger, fear and rage*. 2nd ed. New York: D. Appleton.

———. 1932. *The wisdom of the body*. New York: W. W. Norton.

Carlson, M. 2004. 9/11, Afghanistan, and Iraq: The response of the New York Theatre. *Theatre Survey* 45 (1): 3–17.

Catlin-Jairazbhoy, A. 2004. A Sidi CD? Globalising African-Indian music and the sacred. In *Sidis and scholars: Essays on African Indians*, ed. A. Catlin-Jairazbhoy and E. A. Alpers, 178–211. Lawrenceville, NJ: Red Sea Press.

Chang, M., and F. Leventhal. 1995. Mobilizing battered women: A creative step forward. In *Dance and other expressive art therapies: When words are not enough*, ed. F. J. Levy with J. P. Fried and F. Leventhal, 59–68. New York: Routledge.

Chilivumbo, A. 1969. Some traditional Malawi dances: A preliminary account. Mimeographed.

Christakis, N. A., and P. D. Allison. 2006. Mortality after the hospitalization of a spouse. *New England Journal of Medicine* 354 (7): 719–30.

Chryst, G. 1986. Interview by Effie Mihopoulos. *Salome* 44/45/46:44–48.

Clark, V. A., and S. E. Johnson, eds. 2005. *Kaiso! Writings by and about Katyherine Dunham*. Madison: University of Wisconsin Press.

Cohen-Sandler, R. 2005. *Stressed-out girls: Helping them thrive in the age of pressure*. New York: Viking.

Cole, S. W., M. E. Kemeny, J. L. Fahey, J. A. Zack, and B. D. Naliboff. 2003. Psychological risk factors for HIV pathogenesis: Mediation by the autonomic nervous system. *Biological Psychiatry* 54 (12): 1444–56.

Conraths-Lange, N. 2003. *Pas de deux*: Daughters, mothers, and dance talk. *Medical Problems of Performing Artists* 18 (2): 52–58.

Cooper, K. H. 1970. *The new aerobics*. New York: Bantam.

Coyle, J. T. 2003. Use it or lose it: Do effortful mental activities protect against dementia? *New England Journal of Medicine* 348 (25): 2489–90.

Crapanzano, V. 1973. *The Hamadsha: A study in Moroccan ethnopsychiatry*. Berkeley and Los Angeles: University of California Press.

Cruz, R., and C. R. Berrol, eds. 2004. *Dance/movement therapists in action: A working guide to research options*. Springfield, IL: Charles C. Thomas.

Csikszentmihalyi, M. 1975. *Beyond boredom and anxiety: The experience in work and games*. San Francisco: Jossey-Bass.

Damasio, A. 2003. Looking for Spinoza: Joy, sorrow and the feeling brain. Orlando, FL: Harcourt.

Dancers Forum. 2002. The dancers forum compact for a working artistic relationship between dancers and choreographers. www.nyfa.org/files_uploaded/DancersForum Compact.pdf.

Deans, J. 2001. Black ballerinas dancing on the edge: An analysis of the cultural politics in Delores Browne's and Raven Wilkinson's careers, 1954–1985. EdD diss., Temple University.

DeFrantz, T. 2004. *Dancing revelations: Alvin Ailey's embodiment of African American culture*. New York: Oxford University Press.

Delaney, W. 1982. Dance therapy in evaluation and treatment. In *A clinician's manual on mental health care*, ed. H. S. Moffic and G. L. Adams, 154–60. Menlo Park, CA: Addison-Wesley.

Dell, C. 1970. *A primer for movement description using effort-shape and supplementary concepts*. New York: Dance Notation Bureau.

De Martino, E. 1966. *La terre du remords*. Trans. C. Poncet. Paris: Gallimard. (Orig. pub. 1961.)

De Mille, A. 1960. *To a young dancer: A handbook for dance students, parents, and teachers*. Boston: Little, Brown.

DeNatale, Bob. 2002. Flesh and blood mystery theater. http://home.earthlink. net/~bdenatale/AboutButoh.html.

Dorward, D. C. 1982. *The Igbo "women's war" of 1929: Documents relating to the Aba riots in Eastern Nigeria*. New York: Microform Ltd.

Douglas, M. 1970. *Purity and danger: An analysis of concepts of pollution and taboo*. Harmondsworth, UK: Penguin.

———. 1973. *Natural symbols*. Harmondsworth, UK: Penguin.

Dow, J. 1986. Universal aspects of symbolic healing: A theoretical synthesis. *Current Anthropology* 88 (1): 56–69.

Dowling, J. 2004. Follow the money: Young dance artists confront the discouraging logistics of working in New York now. *Village Voice*, April 20.

Dresser, N. 1996. *Multicultural manners: New rules of etiquette for a changing society*. New York: Wiley.

Drewal, M. T. 1992. *Yoruba ritual: Performers, play, agency*. Bloomington: Indiana University Press.

Duke, L. 2004. We can't look—and can't look away. *Washington Post*, November 21, D1, 3.

Dulicai, D., and M. Berger. 2005. Global dance/movement therapy growth and development. *The Arts in Psychotherapy Special Issue on the International Scope of Arts Therapies* 32 (3): 205–16.

Dunn, A. L., M. H. Trivedi, J. B. Kampert, C. G. Clark, and H. O. Chambliss. 2005. Exercise treatment for depression: Efficacy and dose response. *American Journal of Preventive Medicine* 28 (1): 1–8.

Dunning, J. 1986. Dance: Eleo Pomare Troupe on Mandela theme. *New York Times*, February 24, C13.

———. 1987. Eviction for Erick Hawkins. *New York Times*, May 30, 13.

———. 2004. Past and present, passionately blended. *New York Times*, September 4, A21.

Eley, S. E. 2004. The little company that could. *Dance Teacher*, March, 36–40.

Epel, S., E. H. Blackburn, J. Lin, F. S. Dhabhar, N. E. Adler, J. D. Morrow, and R. M. Cawthon. Accelerated telomere shortening in response to life stress. *Proceedings of the National Academy of Sciences* 101 (49): 1,7312–15.

Exiner, J., and D. Kelynack. 1994. *Dance therapy redefined: A body approach to therapeutic dance*. With N. Aitchison and J. Czulak. Springfield, IL: Charles C. Thomas.

Farrell, S. 1990. *Holding on to the air: An autobiography.* With T. Bentley. New York: Summit Books.

Farrer, C. R. 1976. Play and inter-ethnic communication. In *The anthropological study of play,* ed. D. Lancy and B. A. Tindal, 86–92. Cornwall, NY: Leisure Press.

Fergusson, E. 1931. *Dancing gods: Indian ceremonials of New Mexico and Arizona.* Albuquerque: University of New Mexico Press.

Fernandez, J. 1982. *Bwiti: An ethnography of the religious imagination in Africa.* Princeton, NJ: Princeton University Press.

Fishman, K. D. 2004. *Attitude! Eight young dancers come of age at the Ailey School.* New York: Jeremy P. Tarcher/Penguin.

Fitt, S. S. 1996. *Dance kinesiology.* 2nd ed. Belmont, CA: Wadsworth Publishing.

Forman, J. S. 1983. The effects of an aerobic dance program for women teachers on symptoms of burnout. PhD diss., University of Cincinnati.

Forsyth, S., and P. M. Kolenda. 1966. Competition, cooperation, and group cohesion in the ballet company. *Psychiatry* 29 (2): 123–45.

Fox, K. 1999. The influences of physical activity on mental well-being. *Public Health Nutrition* 2 (3a): 411–18.

Frank, J. E. 1973. *Persuasion and healing: A comparative study of psychotherapy.* Rev. ed. Baltimore: Johns Hopkins University Press.

Frank, Z. 1997. Dance and expressive movement therapy: An effective treatment for a sexually abused man. *American Journal of Dance Therapy* 19 (1): 45–62.

Freud, S. 1955. *Beyond the pleasure principle.* London: Hogarth Press.

Friedman, R. A. 2003. Traversing the mystery of memory. *New York Times,* December 30.

Gailey, H. A. 1970. *The road to Aba: A study of British administrative policy in Eastern Nigeria.* New York: New York University Press.

Gardner, H. 1983. *Frames of mind: A theory of multiple intelligences.* New York: Basic Books.

Gere, D. 2004. *How to make dances in an epidemic: Tracking choreography in the age of AIDS.* Madison: University of Wisconsin Press.

Gold, R. 2001. Confessions of a boy dancer: Running a gantlet of bullying and name-calling. *Dance Magazine* 75 (11): 52.

Goodill, S. W. 2005. *An introduction to medical dance/movement therapy: Health care in motion.* Philadelphia: Jessica Kingsley.

Gordon, S. 1983. *Off balance: The real world of ballet.* New York: Pantheon.

Gottschild, B. D. 2003. *The black dancing body: A geography from coon to cool.* New York: Palgrave Macmillan.

Graham, M. 1985. Martha Graham reflects on her art and a life in dance. *New York Times,* March 31.

Gray, A. E. L. 2001. The body remembers: Dance/movement therapy with an adult survivor of torture. *American Journal of Dance Therapy* 23 (1): 29–43.

Griaule, M. 1965. *Conversations with Ogotemmeli: An introduction to Dogon religious ideas.* London: Oxford University Press.

Gruen, J. 1986. Bruhn on Bruhn. *Dance Magazine* 56 (6): 33.

Guenther, M. G. 1975. The trance dancer as an agent of social change among the farm Bushmen of the Ghanzi district. *Botswana Notes and Records* 7:161–66.

Hackney, P. 2000. *Making connections: Total body integration through Bartenieff Fundamentals.* New York: Routledge.

Hager, B. 1978. *The dancer's world: Problems of today and tomorrow.* Paris: UNESCO Cultural Development Documentary Dossier.

Halpern, R. H. 1981. *Female occupational exhibitionism: An exploratory study of topless and bottomless dancers.* Ann Arbor, MI: University Microfilms.

Halprin, D. 2003. *The expressive body in art and therapy. Working with movement, metaphor and meaning.* London: Jessica Kingsley.

Hamilton, L. 1997. The dancers' health survey: From injury to peak performance. Pt. 2. *Dance Magazine* 71 (2): 60–65.

_____. 1998. *Advice for dancers: Emotional counsel and practical strategies.* San Francisco: Jossey-Bass.

_____. 1999. Coming out in dance: Paths to understanding. *Dance Magazine* 73 (2): 72–75.

Hamilton, L., and W. G. Hamilton. 1994. Occupational stress in classical ballet: The impact in different cultures. *Medical Problems of Performing Artists* 9 (2): 35–38.

Hamilton, L., J. J. Hella, and W. G. Hamilton. 1995. Personality and occupational stress in elite performers. *Medical Problems of Performing Artists* 10 (3): 86–89.

Hanna, J. L. 1970. Discussion of Rod Rodger's session (Dance mobilization as therapy in the inner city; research design). In *Research in Dance: Problems and Possibilities,* 37–42 and 62–63. New York: Postgraduate Center for Mental Health.

_____. 1976. *The anthropology of dance ritual: Nigeria's Ubakala nkwa di iche iche.* Ann Arbor, MI: University Microfilms.

_____. 1978. African dance: Some implications for dance therapy. *American Journal of Dance Therapy* 2 (1): 3–15.

_____. 1979a. Movements toward understanding humans through the anthropological study of dance. *Current Anthropology* 20 (2): 313–39.

_____. 1979b. Toward semantic analysis of movement behavior: Concepts and problems. *Semiotica* 25 (1–2): 77–110.

_____. 1982. Public policy and the children's world: Implications of ethnographic research for desegregated schooling. In *Doing the ethnography of schooling: Educational anthropology in action,* ed. G. D. Spindler, 316–55. New York: Holt, Rinehart and Winston.

_____. 1983. *The performer-audience connection: Emotion to metaphor in dance and society.* Austin: University of Texas Press.

_____. 1984. Towards discovering the universals of dance. *World of Music* 26 (2): 88–103.

_____. 1985. The impact of the critic: Comments from the critics and the criticized. In *Social science and the arts, 1984,* ed. J. Robinson, 141–62. Lanham, MD: University Press of America.

———. 1986a. Interethnic communication in children's own dance, play, and protest. In *Interethnic Communication*, ed. Y. Y. Kim, 176–98. International and Intercultural Communication Annual 10. Newbury Park, CA: Sage Publications.

———. 1986b. Movement in African performance. In *Theatrical movement: A bibliographical anthology*, ed. B. Fleshman, 561–85. Metuchen, NJ: Scarecrow Press.

———. 1987a. Dance and religion (overview). In *The Encyclopedia of Religion*, ed. Mircea Eliade, 203–12. Vol. 4. New York: Macmillan.

———. 1987b. *To dance is human: A theory of nonverbal communication.* Chicago: University of Chicago Press.

———. 1988a. *Dance, sex and gender: Signs of identity, dominance, defiance and desire.* Chicago: University of Chicago Press.

———. 1988b. *Disruptive school behavior: Class, race, and culture.* New York: Holmes and Meier.

———. 1988c. The representation and reality of divinity in dance. *Journal of the American Academy of Religion* 56 (2): 501–26.

———. 1989. African dance frame by frame: Revelation of sex roles through distinctive feature analysis and comments on field research, film, and notation. *Journal of Black Studies* 19 (4): 422–41.

———. 1990a. Advertising with dance. In *Dance: Current selected research*, ed. L. Y. Overby and J. H. Humphrey, 117–36. Vol. 2. New York: AMS Press.

———. 1990b. Anthropological perspectives for dance/movement therapy. *American Journal of Dance Therapy* 12 (2) : 115–26.

———. 1995. The power of dance: Health and healing. *Journal of Alternative and Complementary Medicine* 1 (4): 323–27.

———. 1997. Rasta Thomas: Extraordinary boy next door. *Dance Teacher Now* 19 (1): 65– 72.

———. 1998. Undressing the First Amendment and corseting the striptease dancer. *Drama Review* T158, 42 (2): 38–69.

———. 1999. *Partnering dance and education: Intelligent moves for changing times.* Champaign, IL: Human Kinetics.

———. 2002a. The performing arts world according to Rand: A review of two studies. *Dance/USA Journal* 18 (2–3): 40–42.

———. 2002b. Rasta's quest: Ballet's maverick is still looking for a home. *Dance Magazine* 76 (6): 40–43, 68–69.

———. 2003. Exotic dance adult entertainment: Ethnography challenges false mythology. *City and Society* 15 (2): 165–93.

———. 2004a. Cuba: A little island and a lot of dance. *Dancer*, July, 44–49.

———. 2004b. Cuban dance on street, stage and page. With Ramiro Guerra. *Dance Critics Association News*, Fall, 8–13.

———. 2004c. Social dancing; Dance classes; Performing arts audiences. In *Encyclopedia of recreation and leisure in America*, ed. G. S. Cross, 284–87, 263–65, 105–7. New York: Charles Scribner's Sons.

_____. 2004d. Dance. In *Encyclopedia of the Harlem Renaissance*, ed. C. Wintz and P. Finkelman, 289–93. 2 vols. New York: Routledge.

_____. 2005a. Adult entertainment exotic dance: A guide for planners and policy makers. *Journal of Planning Literature* 20 (2): 116–34.

_____. 2005b. Dance and religion (overview). In *The encyclopedia of religion*, ed. L. Jones, 2, 134–43. 2nd ed. New York: Macmillan.

_____. 2005c. Rasta Thomas, prodigal son. *Dancer*, January, 58–69.

Hanna, J. L., and W. J. Hanna. 1968. Nkwa di iche iche: Dance-plays of Ubakala. *Presence Africaine* 65:13–38.

Hansen, C. 1967. Jenny's toes: Negro shaking dances in America. *American Quarterly* 19:554–63.

Hecker, J. F. C. 1885. *The dancing mania of the Middle Ages*. Trans. B. G. Babington. New York: J. Fitzgerald.

Heinrichs, M. T., T. Baumgartner, C. Kirschbaum, and U. Ehlert. 2003. Social support and oxytocin interact to suppress cortisol and subjective responses to psychosocial stress. *Biological Psychiatry* 54 (12): 1389–98.

Helin, P. 1989. Mental and psychophysiological tension at professional ballet dancers' performances and rehearsals. *Dance Research Journal* 21 (1): 7–14.

Hendin, J., and M. Csikszentmihalyi. 1975. Measuring the flow experience in rock dancing. In *Beyond boredom and anxiety*, ed. M. Csikszentmihalyi, 102–22. San Francisco: Jossey-Bass.

Ho, R. T. 2005. Regaining balance within: Dance movement therapy with Chinese cancer patients in Hong Kong. *American Journal of Dance Therapy* 27 (2): 87–99.

Hoerburger, F. 1965. Folk dance survey. Pt. 1. *Journal of the International Folk Music Council* 17:7–8.

Hoge, C. W., C. A. Castro, S. C. Messer, D. McGurk, D. I. Cotting, and R. L. Koffman. 2004. Combat duty in Iraq and Afghanistan, mental health problems, and barriers to care. *New England Journal of Medicine* 351 (1): 13–22.

Holcomb, J. M. 1977. The effects of dancing and relaxation sessions on stress levels of senior citizens. PhD diss., United States International University.

Horton, R. 1960. *The gods as guests: An aspect of Kalabari religious life*. Lagos: Nigeria Magazine Special Publication.

Howard, J. H. 1983. Pan-Indianism in native American music and dance. *Ethnomusicology* 27 (1): 71–82.

Howes, J., and M. McCormack. 2000. *Dance technique and injury prevention*. 3rd. ed. New York: Routledge.

Hutchinson, A. 1961. *Labanotation: The system for recording movement*. New York: New Directions Book.

Huwyler, J. S. 2002. *The dancer's body: A medical perspective on dance and dance training*. London: Dance Books.

Ice, G., and G. D. James, eds. 2006. *Measuring stress in humans: A practical guide for field research*. New York: Cambridge University Press.

Ilogu, E. 1965. Christianity and Ibo traditional religion. *International Revue of Missions* 54 (215): 335–42.

Insel, T. R., B. S. Gingrich, and L. J. Young. 2001. Oxytocin: Who needs it? *Progress in Brain Research* 133:59–66.

Jackson, A. W., J. R. Morrow Jr., D. W. Hill, and R. K. Dishman. 2004. *Physical activity for health and fitness.* Updated ed. Champaign, IL: Human Kinetics.

Jackson, G. 1978. *Dance as dance: Selected reviews and essays.* Ontario, Canada: Catalyst.

Jackson, P. 2004. *Inside clubbing: Sensual experiments in the art of being human.* New York: Berg.

Jacob, E. 1981. *Dancing: A guide for the dancer you can be.* Reading, MA: Addison-Wesley.

Jones, B., and B. L. Hawes. 1972. *Step it down: Games, plays and stories from the Afro-American heritage.* New York: Harper and Row.

Jowitt, D. 1995. Anna Sokolow. *Dance Magazine* 69 (8): 38–43.

Kapferer, B. A. 1983. *A celebration of demons: Exorcism and the aesthetics of healing in Sri Lanka.* Bloomington: Indiana University Press.

Kealiinohomoku, J. 1969–1970. An anthropologist looks at ballet as a form of ethnic dance. *Impulse: Extensions of Dance,* 24–33.

Keleman, S. 1975. *Living your dying.* New York: Random House.

Kelly, J. 2005. *The great mortality: An intimate history of the Black Death, the most devastating plague of all time.* New York: HarperCollins.

Kelly-Saxenmeyer, A. 2004. Dancing in time. *Backstage.com,* January 7.

Kendall, L. 1985. *Shamans, housewives, and other restless spirits: Women in Korean ritual life.* Honolulu: University of Hawaii Press.

Kern, L. 1981. *An ordered love: Sex roles and sexuality in Victorian utopias: The Shakers, the Mormons, and the Oneida Community.* Chapel Hill: University of North Carolina Press.

Kirkland, G. 1986. *Dancing on my grave.* New York: Doubleday.

Kisselgoff, A. 1982. Forsythe's "Say Bye-Bye" startles and excites. *New York Times,* August 1, H8.

———. 1989. Jones/Zane Company and loss. *New York Times,* March 20, C16.

Kriegsman, A. M. 1987. The Dance Theatre of Harlem: Steps ahead at the Kennedy Center Opera House, Garth Fagan's "Footprints." *Washington Post,* February 15, F1, 10–11.

Laderman, C. 1996. The poetics of healing in Malay shamanistic performances. In *The performance of healing,* ed. C. Laderman and M. Roseman, 115–41. New York: Routledge.

Lambo, T. A. 1965. The place of the arts in the emotional life of the African. *American Society of African Culture Newsletter* 7 (4): 1–6.

Laufer, A. 2003. Psychological growth in the aftermath of terrorist acts. *Palestine-Israel Journal of Politics, Economics and Culture* 10 (4): 30–36.

Lawler, L. B. 1964. *The dance in ancient Greece.* Middletown, CT: Wesleyan University Press.

Lazarus, R. S. 1999. *Stress and emotion: A new synthesis.* New York: Springer.

Lee, R. B. 1967. Trance cure of the !Kung Bushman. *Natural History* 76 (a): 31–37.

Lerman, L. 1984. *Teaching dance to senior adults.* Springfield, IL: Charles C. Thomas.

Lesté, A., and J. Rust. 1990. Effects of dance on anxiety. *American Journal of Dance Therapy* 12 (1): 19–25.

Levanthal, M. B., ed. 1983. *Graduate research and studies in dance/movement therapy 1972–1982.* Compiled by the Council of Graduate Dance/Movement Therapy Educators. Philadelphia: Hahnemann University Press.

Levine, L. W. 1977. *Culture and black consciousness: Afro-American folk thought from slavery to freedom.* New York: Oxford University Press.

Levy, F., ed. 1995. *Dance and other expressive art therapies: When words are not enough.* With J. P. Fried and F. Leventhal. New York: Macmillan.

———. 2005. *Dance movement therapy: A healing art.* Rev. ed. Reston, VA: National Dance Association.

Lopata, H. Z., and J. Noel. 1972. The dance studio: Style without sex. In *Games, sport and power,* ed. G. P. Stone, 184–201. New Brunswick, NJ: Transaction Books.

Lovallo, W. R. 1997. *Stress and health: Biological and psychological interactions.* Thousand Oaks, CA: Sage Publications.

Mackinnon, L. T. 1992. *Exercise and immunology: Current issues in exercise science.* Monograph no. 2. Champaign, IL: Human Kinetics.

Madsen, W. 1973. *Mexican-Americans of South Texas.* 2nd ed. New York: Holt, Rinehart and Winston.

Magill, R. A. 1985. *Motor learning concepts and applications.* Dubuque, IA: William C. Brown.

Manning, P. K., and H. Fabrega Jr. 1973. The experience of self and body: Health and illness in the Chiapas highlands. In *Phenomenological sociology: Issues and applications,* ed. George Psathas, 251–301. New York: Wiley.

Marmot, M. 2004. *The status syndrome: How social standing affects our health and longevity.* New York: Times Books.

Marshall, L. 1962. !Kung Bushman religious beliefs. *Africa* 32: 221–52.

Martin, C., ed. 1986. Life on the floor: Art, sport, and scam: Dance marathons of the twenties and thirties. *New Observations* 39.

———. 1994. *Dance marathons: Performing American culture of the 1920s and 1930s.* Jackson: University Press of Mississippi.

Martinsen, E. W., J. S. Raglin, A. Hoffart, and S. Friis. 1998. Tolerance to intensive exercise and high levels of lactate in panic disorder. *Journal of Anxiety Disorders* 12 (4): 333–42.

Mason, K. C., ed. 1974. *Therapy: Focus on Dance.* Vol. 7. Washington, DC: American Association for Health, Physical Education and Recreation.

Mazo, J. H. 1974. *Dance is a contact sport.* New York: Dutton.

McCarthy, K., A. Brooks, J. Lowell, and L. Zakaras. 2001. *The performing arts in a new era*. Santa Monica, CA: Rand.

McCarthy, K., and K. Jinnett. 2001. *New framework for building participation in the arts*. Santa Monica, CA: Rand.

McDonald, K. A. 1998. Scientists consider new explanations for the impact of exercise on mood. *Chronicle of Higher Education*, August 14, A15–16.

McElroy, A., and P. K. Townsend. 1979. *Medical anthropology in ecological perspective*. 2nd ed. Boulder, CO: Westview Press.

McEwen, B. 2002. *The end of stress as we know it*. Washington, DC: Joseph Henry Press.

McIntyre, M. 1986. Resisting the recognizable. *Washington Post*, June 2, B7.

McKean, P. F. 1979. From purity to pollution: The Balinese Ketjak (monkey dance) as symbolic form in transition. In *The imagination of reality*, ed. A. L. Becker and A. A. Yenogyan, 293–302. Norwood, NJ: Ablex.

McNally, R. J. 2003. *Remembering trauma*. Cambridge, MA: Harvard University Press.

McNees, P. 1987. Diversions: Folk dancing's leaps and bounds: Every night, there's action. *Washington Post*, February 6, C5.

Meek, C. K. 1931. *Tribal studies in northern Nigeria*. London: Kegan Paul, Trench, Trubner.

———. 1937. *Law and authority in a Nigerian tribe*. London: Oxford University Press.

Meekum, B. 2002. *Dance movement therapy*. Thousand Oaks, CA: Sage.

Meyers, M. 1986. Perceptual awareness in integrative movement behavior: The role of integrative movement systems body therapies in motor performance and expressivity. In *The dancer as athlete*, ed. C. G. Shell, 163–86. Champaign, IL: Human Kinetics.

Meyers, M., M. Pierpont, and D. Schnitt. 1986. Body systems. In *Theatrical movement: A bibliographical anthology*, ed. B. Fleshman, 100–14. Metuchen, NJ: Scarecrow Press.

Middleton, J. 1985. The dance among the Lugbara of Uganda. In *Society and the dance*, ed. P. Spencer, 165–82. Cambridge: Cambridge University Press.

Mitchell, J. C. 1956. *The Kalela dance*. Manchester: Manchester University Press for the Rhodes-Livingstone Institute.

Mobbs, D., M. D. Greicius, E. Abdel-Azim, V. Menon, and A. L. Reiss. 2003. Humor modulates the mesolimbic reward centers. *Neuron* 40:1041–48.

Moedano, G. 1972. Los hermanos de la Santa Cuenta: Un culto de crisis de origen Chichimeca. In *Religion en Mesoamerica*. Mesa Redonda, Sociedad Mexicana de Antropologia 12. Ed. Jaime Litvak King and Noemí Castillo. Tejero, Mexico: La Sociedad.

Moffet, H., L. Noreau, E. Parent, and M. Drolet. 2002. Feasibility of an eight-week dance-based exercise program and its effects on locomotor ability of persons with functional class III rheumatoid arthritis. *Arthritis Care and Research* 13 (2): 100–11.

Montoye, H. J. 1984. Exercise and osteoporosis in exercise and health. In *Exercise and health: American Academy of Physical Education papers*, ed. H. M. Eckert and H. J. Montoye, 19–75. No. 17. Champaign, IL: Human Kinetics.

Mooney, J. 1965. *The Ghost-dance religion and the Sioux outbreak of 1890.* Ed. A. F. C. Wallace. Chicago: University of Chicago Press. (Orig. pub. 1896.)

Mora, G. 1963. An historical and sociopsychiatric appraisal of tarantism and its importance in the tradition of psychotherapy of mental disorders. *Bulletin of the History of Medicine* 37:417–39.

Morgan, W. P. 1984. Physical activity and mental health. In *Exercise and health: American Academy of Physical Education Papers,* ed. H. M. Eckert and H. J. Montoye, 132–45. No. 17. Champaign, IL: Human Kinetics.

———. 1985. Affective beneficence of vigorous physical activity. *Medicine and Science in Sports and Exercise* 17 (1): 94–100.

Morley, J. F., and R. I. Morimoto. 2004. Regulation of longevity in *caenorhabditis elegans* by heat shock factor and molecular chaperones. *Molecular Biology of the Cell* 15:657–64.

Munroe, R. L. 1955. *Schools of psychoanalytic thought: An exposition, critique and attempt at integration.* New York: Holt, Rinehart and Winston.

Myers, S. L. 2003. Battlefield aid for soldiers' battered psyches. *New York Times,* June 21.

National Endowment for the Arts. 2003. Arts provide proven benefits to patients and care providers. July 1, 2003. www.nea.gov/news/news03/AIHRelease.html.

Nemetz, L. D. 2004. Being in the body: Finding reconnection after 9/11. *Dance Therapy Association of Australia Quarterly: Moving On* 3 (2): 2–11.

Nichter, M., and M. Lock, eds. 2002. *New horizons in medical anthropology: Essays in honor of Charles Leslie.* New York: Routledge.

Nieman, D. C. 1998. *The exercise-health connection.* Champaign, IL: Human Kinetics.

Nigerian Government. 1930a. *Aba commission of enquiry: Minutes of evidence.*

———. 1930b. *Report of the commission of inquiry appointed to inquire into the disturbances in the Calabar and Owerri Provinces.* December 1929. Sessional paper of the Nigerian Legislative Council, 28.

Njaka, M. E. N. 1974. *Igbo political culture.* Evanston, IL: Northwestern University Press.

Novack, C. 1990. *Sharing the dance: Contact improvisation and American culture.* Madison: University of Wisconsin Press.

Nwabara, S. N. 1965. Igo land: A study in British penetration and the problem of administration, 1860–1930. PhD diss., Michigan State University.

Nwoga, D. I. 1971. The concept and practice of satire among the Igbo. *Conch* 3 (2): 30–45.

O'Connor, D. B., and M. Shimizu. 2002. Sense of personal control, stress and coping style: A cross-cultural study. *Stress and Health* 18:173–83.

Okonkwo, J. I. 1971. Adam and Eve: Igbo marriage in the Nigerian novel. *Conch* 3 (2): 137–51.

Onwuteaka, J. D. 1965. The Aba riot and its relation to the system of indirect rule. *Nigerian Journal of Economic and Social Studies* 7 (3): 273–82.

Ottenberg, P., and S. Ottenberg. 1964. Ibo education and social change. In *Education and politics in Nigeria,* ed. H. N. Weiler, 25–56. Freiburg im Breisgau, Germany: Verlag Rombach.

Overby, L. Y. 1986. A comparison of novice and experienced dancers' imagery ability with respect to their performance on two body awareness tasks. PhD diss., University of Maryland.

Overby, L. Y., and J. H. Humphrey, eds. 1989–. *Dance: Current selected research*. New York: AMS Press.

Paffenbarger, R. Jr., R. T. Hyde, A. L. Wing, and C. Hsien. 1986. Physical activity, all-cause morality, and longevity of college alumni. *New England Journal of Medicine* 314 (10): 605–13.

Panov, V. 1978. *To dance*. New York: Alfred Knopf.

Parks, G. 1986. New lease on Lar. *Dance Magazine* 60 (11): 54–56.

Payne, H., ed. 1992. *Dance movement therapy: Theory and practice*. London: Tavistock/Routledge.

Payne, R. L., and C. L. Cooper. 2001. *Emotions at work: Theory, research and applications for management*. Chichester, UK: Wiley.

Peiss, K. 1986. *Cheap amusements: American working women and leisure in turn-of-the-century New York*. Philadelphia: Temple University Press.

Perham, M. 1937. *Native administration in Nigeria*. London: Oxford University Press.

Perlman, S. G., K. J. Connell, A. Clark, M. S. Robinson, P. Conlon, M. Gech, P. Caldron, J. M. Sinacore. 1990. Dance-based aerobic exercise for rheumatoid arthritis. *Arthritis Care Research* 3 (1): 29–35.

Pierpont, M. 1984. At the edge of education: Naropa. *Dance Magazine* 58 (77): 68–70.

Plevin, M. 2003. Remembering not to forget. *Moving On: Dance Therapy Association of Australia Quarterly Journal* 2 (1): 7–21.

Pollock, M. L., J. H. Wilmore, and S. M. Fox, III. 1984. *Exercise in health and disease: Evaluation and prescription for prevention and rehabilitation*. Philadelphia: W. B. Saunders.

Raglin, J. S. 1997. Anxiolytic effects of physical activity. In *Physical activity and mental health*, ed. W. P. Morgan, 107–26. Washington, DC: Taylor and Francis.

Rand, R. 2004. *Dancing away an anxious mind: A memoir about overcoming panic disorder*. Madison: University of Wisconsin Press.

Ranger, T. O. 1975. *Dance and society in Eastern Africa, 1890–1970: The Beni Ngoma*. Berkeley and Los Angeles: University of California Press.

Raymond, J. 1979. *Transsexual empire*. Boston: Beacon Press.

Reagan, R. 1983. Why I quit the ballet. *Newsweek*, February 14, 11.

Reid, T. R. 2003. Voters could help Denver find its bliss: Anti-stress bill gains support, but council fears ridicule. *Washington Post*, November 2, A3.

Rigby, P. 1966. Dual symbolic classification among the Gogo of Central Tanzania. *Africa* 36 (1): 1–17.

Robben, A. C. G., and M. M. Suárez-Orozco, eds. 2000. *Cultures under siege: Collective violence and trauma*. New York: Cambridge University Press.

Roberts, F. 2004. The sincerest form of Flannery. *New York Times*, February 1. www.nytimes.com/2004/02/01/arts/dance/01ROBE.html

Robson, B. E., and E. Gillies. 1987. Post-performance depression in arts students. *Medical Problems of Performing Artists* 2 (4): 137–41.

Rockwell, I. Nadel. 1984. On stage. *Naropa,* February, 37–38.

———. 1988. Dance: The creative process from a contemplative point of view. In *Dance: Current selected research,* ed. L. Y. Overby and J. H. Humphrey, 187–98. Vol. 1. New York: AMS Press.

———. 2002. Making sense out of modernity. In *New horizons in medical anthropology: Essays in honor of Charles Leslie,* ed. M. Nichter and M. Lock, 111–40. New York: Routledge.

Rohter, L. 2003. A downer of a dance, the tango is in again. *New York Times,* March 8.

Roseman, M. 1991. *Healing sounds from the Malaysian rainforest: Temiar music and medicine.* Comparative Studies of Health Systems and Medical Care 28. Berkeley and Los Angeles: University of California Press.

Rosenkranz, M., W. W. Busse, T. Johnstone, C. A. Swenson, G. M. Crisafi, M. M. Jackson, J. A. Bosch, J. F. Sheridan, and R. J. Davidson. 2005. Neural circuitry underlying the interaction between emotion and asthma symptom exacerbation. *Proceedings of the National Academy of Sciences* 102 (37): 1,3319–24.

Ross, J. 1989. Halprin takes steps for people with AIDS. *Dance Magazine* 63 (4): 9.

Roth, G. 1997. *Sweat your prayers: Movement as spiritual practice.* New York: Jeremy P. Tarcher/Putnam.

Rouget, G. 1985. *Music and trance: A theory of the relations between music and possession.* Trans. and rev. B. Biebuyck. Chicago: University of Chicago Press.

Rovner, S. 1986. Depression and grief: A biological link. *Washington Post,* June 11, health section, 6.

Russell, J. F. 1979. Tarantism. *Medical History* 23 (4): 404–25.

Sachs, M. L., and G. W. Buffone, eds. 1984. *Running as therapy: An integrated approach.* Lincoln: University of Nebraska Press.

Safier, B. 1953. A psychological orientation to dance and pantomime. *Samiksa* 7:236–59.

Samuels, S. 2001. Bringing to light the stresses of war. *New York Times,* December 30, 28, 34.

Sandel, S. L. 1979. Sexual issues in movement therapy with geriatric patients. *American Journal of Dance Therapy* 3 (4): 4–14.

———. 1980. Countertransference stress in the treatment of schizophrenic patients. *American Journal of Dance Therapy* 3 (2): 20–32.

Sangree, W. 1969. Going home to mother: Traditional marriage among the Irigwe, Benue-Plateau State, Nigeria. *American Anthropologist* 71 (6): 1,046–57.

Sapolsky, R. M. 2004. *Why zebras don't get ulcers: An updated guide to stress, stress related diseases, and coping.* 3rd ed. New York: Henry Holt.

Schechner, R. 1973. Drama, script, theatre, and performance. *Drama Review* 17 (3): 5–36.

Scheff, T. J. 1977. The distancing of emotion in ritual with CA comment. *Current Anthropology* 18 (3): 483–505.

Schmais, C. 1985. Healing processes in group dance therapy. *American Journal of Dance Therapy* 8:17–36.

_____. 2004. *The journey of a dance therapy teacher: Capturing the essence of Chace.* Columbia, MD: Marian Chace Foundation of the American Dance Therapy Association.

Schneider, M. 1948. *La danza de espadas y la tarentela. Ensayo musicológico, etnografico y arqueológico sobre los ritos medicinales.* Barcelona: Instituto Espanol de Musicologia.

Schoenfeld, L. 1986. Dance does it. *Dance Magazine* 55 (5): 131.

Schwartz, J. 2004. Always on the job, employees pay with health. in document *New York Times*, September 5, A1, 23.

Selye, H. 1974. *Stress without distress.* Philadelphia: J. B. Lippincott.

_____. 1976. *The stress of life.* New York: McGraw Hill.

Serlin, I. A. 1977. Portrait of Karen: A gestalt-phenomenological approach to movement therapy. *Journal of Contemporary Psychotherapy* 8 (2): 145–53.

_____. 1985. Kinesthetic imagining: A phenomenological study. PhD diss., University of Dallas.

Shell, C. G., ed. 1986. *The dancer as athlete.* 1984 Olympic scientific congress proceedings. Vol. 80. Champaign, IL: Human Kinetics.

Shorter, E. 1982. *A short history of women's bodies.* New York: Basic Books.

Siegel, E. V. 1984. *Movement therapy: The mirror of ourselves: A psychoanalytic approach.* New York: Human Sciences Press.

Siegel, M. 1977. *Watching the dance go by.* Boston: Houghton Mifflin.

Signorile, M. 1997. A troubling double standard. *New York Times*, op-ed, August 16.

Silver, J. A. 1981. Therapeutic aspects of folk dance: Self concept, body concept, ethnic distancing and social distancing. PhD diss., University of Toronto.

Singer, A. J. 2005. "Hidden treasures, hidden voices": An ethnographic study into the use of movement and creativity in developmental work with war affected refugee children (Serbia 2001–2). Paper presented at Dance Ethnography Forum, Leicester, UK, January 29.

Skye, F. D., O. J. Christensen, and J. T. England. 1989. A study of the effects of a culturally-based dance education model on identified stress factors in American Indian college women. *Journal of American Indian Education* 29 (1): 26–31.

Smith, E. L., and R. Serfass, eds. 1981. *Exercise and aging: The scientific bases.* Hillside, NJ: Enslow Publishers.

Smith, R. E., J. T. Ptacek, and E. Patterson. 2000. Moderator effects of cognitive and somatic trait anxiety on the relation between life stress and physical injuries. *Journal of Anxiety, Stress, and Coping* 13:269–88.

Smith, T. M. 2003. *Raising the barre: The geographic, financial and economic trends of nonprofit dance companies.* Research Division Report 44. Washington, DC: National Endowment for the Arts.

Snyder, C. R., ed. 2001. *Coping with stress: Effective people and processes.* New York: Oxford University Press.

Solomon, R., J. Solomon, and S. C. Minton, eds. 2005. Preventing dance injuries. 2nd ed. Champaign, IL: Human Kinetics.

Solway, D. 1986. In a dancer's world, the inexorable foe is time. *New York Times*, June 8, C1, 8.

Sommer, S. R. 1983. Night in the slammer. *Village Voice*, January 18, 29–31, 106.

Spencer, P. 1985. Dance as antithesis in the Samburu discourse. In *Society and the dance*, ed. P. Spencer, 140–64. Cambridge: Cambridge University Press.

Squires. S. 2001. For success, limit the stress. *Washington Post*, December 18, F3.

Stein, M. B. 2005. Sweating away the blues: Can exercise treat depression? *American Journal of Preventive Medicine* 28 (1): 140–41.

Stewart, O. C. 1980. The Ghost Dance. In *Anthropology on the great plains*, ed. W. R. Wood and M. Liberty, 179–87. Lincoln: University of Nebraska Press.

Stone, M. 1975. *At the sign of midnight: The Concheros dance cult of Mexico*. Tucson: University of Arizona Press.

Stoop, N. M. 1984. The Canadian cosmopolitan: Montreal's Brian Macdonald. *Dance Magazine* 58 (4): 62–65.

Strik, J. J. M. H., J. Denollet, R. Lousberg, and A. Honig. 2003. Comparing symptoms of depression and anxiety as predictors of cardiac events and increased health care consumption after myocardial infarction. *Journal of American College of Cardiology* 42 (10): 1801–7.

*Sydney Morning Herald*. 2003. October 23.

Tamuno, T. N. 1966. Before British police in Nigeria. *Nigeria* 89:102–26.

Taylor, P. 1999. *Private domain*. Pittsburgh: University of Pittsburgh Press.

Temin, C. 1982. The master builder. *Ballet News* 3 (11): 16–18, 20, 41.

Ten Raa, E. 1969. The moon as a symbol of life and fertility in Sandawe thought. *Africa* 39:24–53.

Thomas, H. 2003. *The body, dance and cultural theory*. New York: Palgrave Macmillan.

Thompson, B. 2004. For Neve Campbell, a painful stretch. *Washington Post*, B1, 7.

Thornton, R. 1981. Demographic antecedents of a revitalization movement, population change, population size, and the 1890 Ghost Dance. *American Sociological Review* 46 (1): 88–96.

Tipton, C. I., ed. 2003. *Exercise physiology: People and ideas*. New York: Oxford University Press.

Toates, F. 1995. *Stress: Conceptual and biological aspects*. New York: Wiley.

Turner, R. J., B. Wheaton, and D. A. Lloyd. 1995. The epidemiology of social stress. *American Sociological Review* 60 (2): 104–05.

Turner, V. 1974. *Dramas, fields, and metaphor: Symbolic action in human society*. Ithaca, NY: Cornell University Press.

Uchendu, V. C. 1965. *The Igbo of Southeast Nigeria*. New York: Holt, Rinehart and Winston.

Umunna, I. 1968. Igbo names and the concept of death. *African Scholar* 1 (1): 28.

Van Allen, J. 1972. "Sitting on a man": Colonialism and the lost political institutions of Igbo women. *Canadian Journal of African Studies* 6 (2): 165–81.

Verghese J., R. B. Lipton, M. J. Katz, C. B. Hall, C. A. Derby, M. J. Katz, A. F. Ambrose, M. Sliwinski, and H. Buschke. 2003. Leisure activities and the risk of dementia in the elderly. *New England Journal of Medicine*, 348 (25): 2508–16.

Vincent, L. M. 1979. *Competing with the sylph: Dancer and the pursuit of the ideal body form*. New York: Andrews and McMeel.

Vogel, M. 1986. Fit for work: Do on-the-job wellness programs really pay off? *Washington Post*, July 23, health section, 10–13.

Wallach, M. 1989. Bill T. Jones/Arnie Zane and Co. brave the waters. *New York City Tribune*, March 15.

Wampold, B. E. 2001. *The great psychotherapy debate: Models, methods and findings*. Mahwah, NJ: Lawrence Erlbaum Associates.

Wang, L., X. Wang, W. Wang, C. Chen, A. G. Ronnennberg, W. Guang, A. Huang, Z. Fang, T. Zang, and X. Xu. 2004. Stress and dysmenorrhoea: a population based prospective study. *Occupational and Environmental Medicine* 61:1021–26.

*Washington Post*. 1980. June 25.

*Washington Post*. 1983. Stats. April 26, B7.

Weisbrod, J. 1974. Body movement therapy and the visually-impaired person. In *Focus on Dance*. Vol. 7 of *Dance Therapy*, ed. K. C. Mason, 49–52. Washington, DC: American Association for Health, Physical Education and Recreation.

Weston, E. 1982. *A Report: Conference on career transition for dancers*. New York. Hollywood, CA: Actors' Equity Association.

White, D. 1982. *Update Dance/USA*, 2 (5): 2

White, K. 2006. Making it work. *Pointe* 7 (1): 58–59.

Williams, D. 1968. The dance of the Bedu moon. *African Arts* 2 (1): 18–21.

Williams, M. D. 1974. *Community in a black Pentecostal church: An anthropological study*. Pittsburgh: University of Pittsburgh Press.

Wilson, A. A. 1991. Rehearsals in the anthropology of performance and the performance of anthropology: Ritual, reflexivity, and healing in a dance by men challenging AIDS. MA thesis, University of Southern California.

Wilson, M. 1954. Nyakyusa ritual and symbolism. *American Anthropologist* 56:228–41.

Wilson, R. S., D. A. Evans, J. L. Bienias, C. F. Mendes de Leon, J. A. Schneider, and D. A. Bennett. 2003. Proneness to psychological distress is associated with risk of Alzheimer's disease. *Neurology* 61 (1): 1479–85.

Wittstein I. S., D. R. Thiemann, J. A. C. Lima, K. L. Baughman, S. P. Schulman, G. Gerstenblith, C. Wu, J. J. Rade, T. J. Bivalacqua, and H. C. Champion. 2005. Neurohumoral features of myocardial stunning due to sudden emotional stress. *New England Journal of Medicine* 352 (6): 539–48.

Wolpe, J. 1958. *Psychotherapy by reciprocal inhibition*. Stanford, CA: Stanford University Press.

Yamaguchi, K., K. Toda, and Y. Hayashi. 2003. Effects of stressful training on human brain threshold. *Stress and Health* 19:9–15.

Yusuf, S., S. Hawken, S. Ôunpuu, T. Dans, A. Avezum, F. Lanas, M. McQueen, A. Budaj, P. Pais, J. Varigos, L. Lisheng. 2004. Effect of potentially modifiable risk factors associated with myocardial infarction in 52 countries (the Interheart study): Case-control study. *Lancet*. 364 (9438): 937–52.

Zimmerman, E. 2003. Your brain on stress: An unfocused picture. *New York Times*, July 20, BU 12.

# Index

~

# About the Author

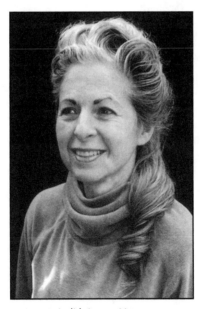

*Judith Lynne Hanna*

Judith Lynne Hanna (PhD, Columbia), a senior research scholar in the Department of Dance at the University of Maryland, College Park, and a consultant in the arts, education, health, public policy, and the First Amendment protection of dance, practices an anthropology that interweaves multidisciplinary theory, research, and application. As a dancer and researcher for over half a century, she has examined dance in its many manifestations and locations, from villages and cities in Africa to children's playgrounds and theaters in America. Her work has been published in thirteen countries and in several languages. She is author of *To Dance Is Human: A Theory of Nonverbal Communication* and *Dance, Sex and Gender: Signs of Identity, Dominance, Defiance and Desire* (both University of Chicago Press), *The Performer-Audience Connection: Emotion to Metaphor in Dance and Society* (University of Texas Press), *Disruptive School Behavior: Class, Race and Culture* (Holmes & Meier), *Partnering Dance and Education: Intelligent Moves for Changing Times* (Human Kinetics), and coauthor of *Urban Dynamics in Black Africa* (Aldine). She has published over three hundred scholarly and other articles in the *New York Times*, the *Washington Post*, *Dance Magazine*, *Stagebill*, and *Dancer*, among other publications. She has taught and lectured at numerous universities in the United States and abroad. Her work on dance and health has appeared in *American Journal of Dance Therapy*, *Dance Teacher*, and *Journal of Alternative and Complementary Medicine*, and she has addressed the Postgraduate Center for Mental Health; the Johns Hopkins University Public Health Program; Uniformed Services University of Health Sciences, School of Medicine; and the National Symposium on Pain.